T0227744

AIDS and Community-Based Drug Intervention Programs: Evaluation and Outreach

AIDS and Community-Based Drug Intervention Programs: Evaluation and Outreach

Dennis G. Fisher, PhD
Richard Needle, PhD
Editors

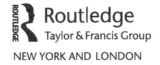

Routledge
Taylor & Francis Group

NEW YORK AND LONDON

AIDS and Community-Based Drug Intervention Programs: Evaluation and Outreach has also been published as *Drugs & Society,* Volume 7, Numbers 3/4 1993.

First published 1993 by The Haworth Press, Inc.

This edition published 2013 by Routledge
605 Third Avenue, New York, NY 10017
4 Park Square, Milton Park, Abingdon, Oxon OX14 4RN

Routledge is an imprint of the Taylor & Francis Group, an informa business

Copyright © 1993 Taylor & Francis

All rights reserved. No part of this book may be reprinted or reproduced or utilised in any form or by any electronic, mechanical, or other means, now known or hereafter invented, including photocopying and recording, or in any information storage or retrieval system, without permission in writing from the publishers.

Notice:
Product or corporate names may be trademarks or registered trademarks, and are used only for identification and explanation without intent to infringe.

Library of Congress Cataloging-in-Publication Data

AIDS and community-based drug intervention programs : evaluation and outreach / Dennis G. Fisher, Richard Needle, editors.
    p. cm.
    Published also as v. 7, no.3/4 1993, of Drugs & Society.
    Includes bibliographical references.
    ISBN 1-56024-510-7 (h : alk. paper).–ISBN   1-56023-050-9 (pp. : alk. paper)
    1. AIDS (Disease)–United States–Prevention. 2. Intravenous drug abuse–United States. I. Fisher, Dennis G. II. Needle, Richard.
    [DNLM: 1. Acquired Immunodeficiency Syndrome–prevention & control–United States–congresses. 2. Acquired Immunodeficieny Syndrome–epidemiology–United States–congresses. 3. Substance Abuse–prevention & control–United States–congresses. 4. Community Mental Health Services–United States–congresses. 5. Epidemiologic Methods–congresses. W1 DR514E v. 7 no.3/4 1993 / WD 308 A2877357 1993]
RA644.A25A343 1993
362.1'969792'00973–dc20
DNLM/DLC
for Library of Congress   93-23471
                                                       CIP

ISBN 13: 978-1-56024-510-0 (hbk)

AIDS and Community-Based Drug Intervention Programs: Evaluation and Outreach

CONTENTS

An Office-Based AIDS Prevention Program for High Risk Drug Users   **205**
     Jon Liebman, MS
     Nina Mulia, MPH

ABOUT THE EDITORS

Dennis G. Fisher, PhD, is Associate Professor and Director of the Center for Alcohol and Addiction Studies at the University of Alaska Anchorage. He was a National Institute on Drug Abuse Epidemiology and Statistics Fellow at the University of California, Los Angeles. The first field representative for the Drug Abuse Division of the Joint Commission on Accreditation of Hospitals, Dr. Fisher was also the previous program evaluation supervisor for the Bureau of Drug Abuse of the State of Ohio.

Richard Needle, PhD, received his doctorate from the University of Maryland and his MPH degree from the University of Minnesota. He was Professor of Family Social Science and Public Health at the University of Minnesota from 1978 until he took a position at NIDA in 1990. In 1983-4, he was on sabbatical from the University of Minnesota, working at the Centers for Disease Control. In September 1992, he became Chief of the Community Research Branch at NIDA.

Preface

The AIDS Prevention Symposium, co-sponsored by the University of Alaska Anchorage, Center for Alcohol and Addiction Studies and the National Institute on Drug Abuse (NIDA), was planned to coincide with a meeting of NIDA-supported Cooperative Agreement for AIDS Community-Based Outreach / Intervention researchers. The Symposium *Proceedings* presented in this volume trace the conceptual, methodological, empirical, and policy-related programmatic developments of the NIDA National AIDS Demonstration Research (NADR) and Cooperative Agreement (CA) projects. They contribute in a significant way to the cumulative literature on these projects published in refereed periodicals, books, and proceedings from NIDA-sponsored NADR national meetings.[1]

Programmatically, both NADR and CA were designed to support development, implementation, and evaluation of community-based interventions targeted to preventing the spread of Human Immunodeficiency Virus (HIV) infection among injection drug users (IDUs), other drug users at high risk for HIV infection, and sexual partners of IDUs. Over 40 communities took part in the NADR project, which began in 1987 and ended in 1992, and 17 sites are currently involved in the CA project, which began in September of 1990. Between 1987 and 1982, the NADR project recruited 45,533 IDUs and sexual partners; between September 1990 and February 1993, the CA project recruited 6,562 IDUs and crack users. Considerable numbers of researchers/investigators, in addition to those involved

[Haworth co-indexing entry note]: "Preface." Needle, Richard. Co-published simultaneously in *Drugs & Society* (The Haworth Press, Inc.) Vol. 7, No. 3/4, 1993, pp. xvii-xxiv; and: *AIDS and Community-Based Drug Intervention Programs: Evaluation and Outreach* (ed: Dennis G. Fisher, and Richard Needle) The Haworth Press, Inc., 1993, pp. xvii-xxiv. Multiple copies of this article/chapter may be purchased from The Haworth Document Delivery Center [1-800-3-HAWORTH; 9:00 a.m. - 5:00 p.m. (EST)].

Copyright © 1993 by Taylor & Francis

in the NADR and CA project and this Symposium, have taken responsibility for developing and implementing community-based programs to prevent the spread of HIV among injection drug users and other populations at high risk for HIV infection.

Much has been learned about recruiting hidden populations, retaining them in intervention activities, and promoting risk reduction behavior. Most community-based programs have relied on field stations in the communities and neighborhoods most greatly affected by the twin epidemics of HIV and drug abuse. Indigenous outreach workers serve as a link between the program and the community. Their presence promotes acceptance of the program and encourages participation in HIV antibody testing, pre- and posttest counseling, and risk reduction education. In addition to recruiting at-risk populations, outreach workers answer questions about HIV and AIDS, distribute condoms and bleach, and provide referrals to other programs and services.[2] The continued presence of outreach workers in the community has been helpful in maintaining contact with at-risk populations and facilitating follow-up of clients.

Risk reduction sessions take the form of individually oriented intervention strategies organized around providing information about risk to self and others, and rely on counseling strategies to facilitate behavior change among the at-risk population. Empirically, it has been demonstrated that these community-based risk reduction and prevention programs are effective in influencing individuals to adopt lower-risk drug use and needle-sharing behaviors and to take advantage of services such as HIV antibody testing, counseling, and drug treatment. Some of the papers in this collection discuss the results of studies comparing different behavior change intervention models.

Since these programs have begun, no single theoretical model has emerged as a key to risk reduction. However, it is clear from the presentations at this Symposium that attention is increasingly being devoted to the adaptation of theoretical perspectives into population-specific approaches to changing behavior. Most of the projects have adopted a psychosocial perspective related to behavior change; more recently, researchers are relying on more sociological/anthropological theories. Over time, an applied research strategy has evolved utilizing the methodologies of epidemiology, ethnography, and evaluation, which have provided a framework for the sampling process, the monitoring of HIV-related risk-taking behaviors among out-of-treatment, non-institutionalized drug-using populations, and the assessment of the efficacy of interventions.

McCoy, Rivers, and Khoury, and Williams and Johnson describe different conceptual perspectives and related research strategies for gaining a better understanding of HIV and drug use and for developing interventions for efficacy testing. McCoy et al. present a public health model that has emerged from their research, discuss empirical data from their NADR experiences, and provide recommendations for future interventions. They also provide a historical overview of the NADR project, calling attention to the commonalities in protocols across programs as well as examining potentially significant differences between programs in research paradigms, enthusiasm for HIV testing, and allocation of resources for different components of programmatic interventions. Findings from their study comparing postintervention changes in AIDS-related risk behaviors, particularly related to drug use, between a standard and an enhanced intervention indicate that no differences were observed between the two interventions. The field is currently examining this issue; CA researchers have learned a great deal from the NADR project about methodology, measurement, and the design of intervention strategies.

The social network perspective, a relatively recently developed paradigm, guides the work of a number of CA sites. Williams and Johnson discuss this model, providing invaluable insight into the potential of this theoretical perspective, as well as accompanying research methodologies, to address unanswered questions about HIV infection among injection drug users. Understanding patterns in the spread of HIV infection, they tell us, particularly in areas where prevalence rates have stabilized, may require studying networks of users and the boundaries between these networks to estimate the likelihood of change in HIV rates. Williams and Johnson's ethnographic study of injection drug users indicates that much remains to be learned about the network structure of IDUs, including dyadic, triadic, and large-group patterns of use. This knowledge will be useful in developing more structured interventions that target networks, rather than individuals, within groups that share certain behavioral patterns.

A number of presenters examine the complex methodological issues that arise in community-based research focusing on hidden populations of drug users. Developing techniques to sample, access, and interview street addicts present a number of methodological challenges. In a conceptual article, Booth et al. rely on examples from their field work to examine the potential contributions of combining qualitative and quantitative research approaches. Booth and other presenters describe field-based applied research techniques that recognize the unique characteristics of the target population and the setting in which the research is conducted. At the same time, they remain consistent with standards of research methodology that require limiting any biases in the study design that could lead to the uninterpretability of data.

Other presenters discuss sampling techniques used to recruit out-of-treatment crack and injection drug users for studies related to monitoring of the behaviors and serostatus of drug addicts. Watters (Watters, along with Biernacki, has described the strategy of targeted sampling)[3] presents an overview of several sampling strategies and focus on the targeted strategy implemented throughout the CA project (which allows investigators to refine or expand the concept of targeted sampling for operationalization within their local areas). Robles, Colón, and Freeman describe a random sampling strategy and recruiting of participants from copping areas in San Juan, Puerto Rico. Copping areas, according to the authors, provide drug users a social context in which to interact and engage in drug-buying and drug-using routines, and thus constitute a setting in which drug users can be identified and approached.

Trotter and Potter discuss the value of using a cognitive anthropology research method called "pile sorts" to evaluate drug and HIV prevention programs. They describe the application of the pile sort technique to explore basic risk as part of their efforts to evaluate the impact of an intervention program for Navajo reservation youth. Their work has great relevance for understanding how to identify and assess culturally defined phenomena that influence behavioral patterns, and may guide the development of culturally sensitive interventions for the at-risk populations involved in the

CA project. The collection of data relevant to HIV risk behaviors in the target populations provides a basis for developing and targeting interventions. While all sites have relied on a common core instrument for data collection in the NADR and CA projects, some presenters focused on selected populations at risk for HIV infection. Chitwood, Rivers, Comerford, and McBride present data on risk behavior and HIV prevalence in a sample of White, non-Hispanic, and African American IDUs in Miami, Florida. Another population whose HIV-related risk behavioral patterns have heretofore received little attention is Native Americans, including Alaska Natives. Fisher, Cagle, and Wilson report a number of findings that have implications for preventing the spread of HIV in Alaska; they note that there is a west coast influence on drug use in Alaska and that, among Alaska Native injectors, women outnumber men. It is hoped that in the future, a clearer understanding of risk behavior characteristics in sub-groups of high-risk populations will facilitate the application of theoretical models to the development of risk reduction interventions.

Rhodes and Humfleet, and Liebman and Mulia report on their prevention programs in Long Beach and Philadelphia, respectively. The Rhodes and Humfleet model is currently being considered for adoption by many State agencies as a result of a NIDA-sponsored technology transfer project that includes training sessions on program implementation. Their model uses a goal-oriented counseling and peer support approach to reduce HIV risks among drug users who are not in treatment.

Deren, Beardsley, Tortu, Davis, and Clatts and Stevens, Erickson, and Estrada report on their studies with women. Deren and colleagues discuss empirical data from their study on behavior change among female injection drug users and sexual partners of IDUs at high risk for HIV infection. Their postintervention findings suggest that both female IDUs and sexual partners can significantly reduce their risk behaviors. They, like other researchers, call for additional research, more focused and targeted interventions, and increased attention to the context of the lives of the target populations—specifically, the social and economic environments. Stevens et al. make this same point based on their study of female sexual partners of injection drug users. They conclude that a single intervention strategy will not be equally effective for all female sexual partners; the intervention must be targeted to the needs of the individual. It is also becoming increasingly clear that intervention design must take into account the HIV seroprevalence rates in the target community.

Presenters at the Symposium also addressed difficult philosophical and practical issues related to program implementation and measures of intervention effectiveness. Ongoing discussion in these projects has centered around the balance between research and practice, an issue that has implications for staff, clients, and overall programmatic progress. Kotranski's paper on the philosophical, substantive, and practical issues involved in conducting a research project with a large public service outreach and education component defines crucial ethical dilemmas that have faced research and service communities since the inception of HIV prevention programs. Changes in the cumulative nature of the research, the various funding mechanisms for programs, ecologies of HIV risk in communities, and progress in the science related to prevention programs and behavior change require continuous attention. These fundamental issues are complex, and programmatic efforts to resolve them have varied. Kotranski offers one valuable perspective.

Another philosophical issue confronting researchers in the NADR and CA projects centers around HIV testing and contact tracing. Smereck reviews strategies from around the country and discusses policy and programmatic implications. The reader will find Smereck's article most interesting and provocative.

Clearly, great progress has been made in planning, implementing, and evaluating community-based prevention programs. It is equally clear that the research community must adapt its paradigms and experiment with a variety of interventions if it hopes to resolve the unanswered questions about HIV and drug use and meet the enormous challenge of preventing further HIV infection in the communities already devastated by this unrelenting epidemic.

Presenters at this Symposium and researchers around the country have helped us better understand that communities vary in their ecologies of drug- and HIV-related risk behaviors, their HIV seroprevalence, and their capacity to mobilize for prevention services. Behavioral heterogeneity characterizes the patterns of individuals within communities; HIV risk behaviors and seroprevalence rates vary by gender, race/ethnicity, and characteristics of drug user contact networks. Risk behaviors related to drug use and needle sharing take on meaning in a social context and most often are undertaken with others–within dyads, triads, and even larger networks of drug users. Future prevention activities should be developed that reflect the community ecology–the epidemiology, ethnography, and behavioral heterogeneity of subgroups of at-risk populations. Interventions should be more clearly targeted to subgroups of high-risk populations, be theoretically driven, and give great attention to measurement issues related to behavior change. We must be able to interpret change and understand groups that do not alter their behaviors.

Progress to date reflects the enormous contributions of the larger professional community–both researchers and practitioners–as well as the presenters at this Symposium who are working to advance the field in the area of prevention. The accompanying bibliographies well illustrate the seminal contributions of the many other investigators in the field of AIDS research, particularly related to prevention programs for injection drug users and their sexual partners.

It has been my privilege to have helped plan this important Symposium and to have given the summary and closing remarks. In addition, I have had the rare combined honor of being a NADR grantee while I was at the University of Minnesota through 1990, prior to joining Dr. Barry Brown at the CRB; NIDA's Principal Investigator on the CA project since it began in 1990; and, currently, the Community Research Branch Chief. The NADR project, from inception through finalization, reflected the enthusiasm and commitment of Drs. George Beschner and Barry Brown, former Branch Chiefs in the Community Research Branch. Dr. Brown played a crucial role in the formulation and implementation of the CA project. All the NADR investigators and CA grantees have worked extraordinarily hard to contribute both to the science and the practice of HIV prevention. Preventing the spread of this epidemic continues to be our highest priority.

Finally, I would be remiss if I did not acknowledge the contributions to NADR and CA of the competent, professionally committed group of NIDA's Community Research Branch Project Officers–

Rebecca Ashery, Helen Cesari, Susan Coyle, Jeanette Johnson, Al Mata, Arnold Mills, Ro Nemeth-Coslett, Gary Palsgrove, Bill Weddington, and Gloria Weissman.

Richard Needle, PhD

NOTES

1. *Community-Based AIDS Prevention: Studies of Intravenous Drug Users and Their Sexual Partners.* (1989). (Proceedings from the First Annual NADR National Meeting, DHHS Publication No. ADM 91-1752.) Washington, DC: U.S. Government Printing Office. *Community-Based AIDS Prevention Among Intravenous Drug Users and Their Sexual Partners: The Many Faces of HIV Disease.* (1990). (Papers Presented at the Second Annual NADR National Meeting.) Bethesda, MD: Nova Research Company.

2. Ashery, R.S. (1992). *Program Development for Community AIDS Outreach* (NIDA Clinical Report Series; DHHS Publication No. ADM-92-1776.) Washington, DC: U.S. Government Printing Office.

3. Watters, J., & Biernacki, P. (1989). Targeted sampling: Options for the study of hidden populations. *Social Problems*, 36, 416-430.

Balancing Prevention Research and Service

Lynne Kotranski, PhD

SUMMARY. A major purpose of public health service and research demonstration projects is to develop models, interventions, or programs geared toward a particular problem. At the same time, these projects need to be structured so that the research design allows for the collection of valid and reliable data that can be used to test the efficacy of the program. The purpose of this paper is to discuss the balance that must be obtained between rigorous research and the ongoing demands of providing services to a target population that is at high risk for contracting and/or transmitting HIV. The paper discusses the day-to-day issues that arise and strategies that have been developed to respond to them.

The purpose of this paper is to discuss the need to balance prevention research and service in demonstration programs. The points

Lynne Kotranski is Vice President for Research and Evaluation at the Philadelphia Health Management Corporation and Co-Principal Investigator of both the NIDA-funded NADR (DA04841) and Cooperative Agreement (DA06919) Programs in Philadelphia.

The author gratefully acknowledges the contributions of PHMC's AIDS outreach workers, health educators, interviewers, and research staff for their insightful observations.
Correspondence may be addressed to the author at: 260 South Broad Street, 20th Floor, Philadelphia, PA 19102.

[Haworth co-indexing entry note]: "Balancing Prevention Research and Service." Kotranski, Lynne. Co-published simultaneously in *Drugs & Society* (The Haworth Press, Inc.) Vol. 7, No. 3/4, 1993, pp. 1-12; and: *AIDS and Community-Based Drug Intervention Programs: Evaluation and Outreach* (ed: Dennis G. Fisher, and Richard Needle) The Haworth Press, Inc., 1993, pp. 1-12. Multiple copies of this article/chapter may be purchased from The Haworth Document Delivery Center [1-800-3-HAWORTH; 9:00 a.m. - 5:00 p.m. (EST)].

Copyright © 1993 by Taylor & Francis

1

to be discussed deal with the realities of trying to implement a research project that has a large service component or attempting to operate a service project that has a large research component. The balance between service and research is an important subject because it underlies some of the basic philosophical issues with which we have to deal, such as whether it is ethical to withhold treatment (whether that treatment involves information, services, and/or medications) from a study population that needs the treatment. There is also a basic substantive issue about the focus of a project that has both service and research components. Any one project cannot be all things to all people and a decision has to be made as to whether the primary focus is research or service. Third, there are practical issues, those that have to be faced every day; in particular, how do you keep a multitude of divergent activities going along on a day-to-day basis and still meet the project and funder requirements?

The discussion to follow is based primarily on the experiences we have had in Philadelphia over the past five years as both a National AIDS Demonstration Research Project (NADR) and Cooperative Agreement site (see *References*). In addition to our ongoing experiences, interviews and focus groups were held with both service staff (health educators, outreach workers) and research staff (senior researchers and interviewers) in order to further identify the issues that are presented here.

BACKGROUND: CONTEXTUAL CHARACTERISTICS

As a starting point in discussing the balance between service and research, it is important to specify the context in which a project is implemented and operational. We have all discussed a need in our own analysis of the research findings to include contextual variables or those characteristics of the larger environment in which our project operates and which can have an independent influence on project effectiveness. Similarly, there are other contextual variables which affect the nature of our projects and how smoothly they operate, and these contextual variables have to be considered when discussing a project's ability to balance prevention or service and research activities.

These contextual characteristics include: (a) the *purpose* of the grant program which funds the project; (b) the *city* in which the program is implemented; (c) the specific *neighborhood* in which services are being provided; (d) the *organization* or agency implementing the project; (e) the *number* of other *sites* involved; and (f) the *resources* that are available and how they can be allocated.

First, there is the purpose of the project. Our current project Cooperative Agreement follows on the heels of the NADR service demonstration program, which has previously been described in this volume. There are currently sixteen (16) projects funded under the Cooperative Agreement for Community Based Monitoring and AIDS Prevention Research. The NADR and Cooperative Agreement grant programs are somewhat different. The former was more service-oriented and the latter is more research-oriented. The purpose of the Cooperative Agreement is to monitor the characteristics of drug users and drug activity as well as testing the efficacy of various types of enhanced interventions across all program sites.

In addition to the purpose of the grant program, a second contextual variable is the city in which a program is being implemented. For example, Philadelphia and New York are very different from Tucson and Dayton, not the least of the differences being the Human Immunodeficiency Virus (HIV) prevalence rate, characteristics of drug users, the actual number of drug users, and the existence of other programs in the city. These characteristics impact on what a program can and cannot do both ethically and politically.

A third contextual variable–the characteristics of the specific neighborhood in which outreach and recruiting takes place–can impose pressures which mandate that staff reevaluate or modify project requirements. There are very real political constraints which are unique to certain neighborhoods and cities. We have oftentimes been told by leaders in certain communities in Philadelphia that we have to "give something back to the neighborhood" and some communities will demand this more than others. Therefore, project outreach cannot function simply as a recruitment mechanism and outreach workers cannot just be recruiters. The outreach workers need to be seen as people who will give something back to the community. Oftentimes, this involves being present, being willing to listen, being caring and giving out condoms and bleach and–even though they are not supposed to–making referrals for those individuals who need assistance from social service agencies or drug abuse treatment programs.

A fourth contextual variable that mediates between service and research is the organization that actually implements the program. There are many differences between university-based settings, private non-profit organizations, profit-making organizations as well as governmental agencies. In Philadelphia, Philadelphia Health Management Corporation has as its mission to engage in service and research/evaluation programs which benefit the public health. We have a Board of Directors which feels very strongly that we should not just be doing research or just collecting information. Other organizations don't necessarily have those constraints, have a different mission and history, and can operate differently.

Another fifth contextual variable, is the number of sites that are involved in a grant program. There is somewhat more flexibility on single site or two site programs in comparison with a multi-site program. The reason for this is that the more sites you have, and the more you want to do comparisons across sites, the more there will be restrictions placed on sites; this can lead to too much homogenization. Accordingly, national level data may not be as useful as for developing national programs because programs will need to be implemented based on what makes sense on a local level; local data are best suited for that.

A final contextual variable, and one which is extremely important in affecting one's ability to balance research and service, is the resources that are available for a program. The extent of available monetary resources affects how many outreach workers you have, how many health educators you can afford, and determines one's flexibility in enhancing the project's service activities while also meeting the requirements of experimental research design. For example, the limited service resources of the Cooperative Agreement has restricted individual projects' ability to continue to engage in the level of outreach available under the NADR program.

IMPACT OF PROJECT REQUIREMENTS: PROJECT NEEDS VERSUS STAFF NEEDS

In addition to the above contextual variables, there are day-to-day issues that arise and which must be addressed as we balance service and prevention research. One of the characteristics of social science research is that researchers are often forced to be creative and formulate workable solutions. The issues and examples discussed below serve to illustrate how we balance service and research.

To a large extent, the basic philosophical and ethical issues about the need for control and experimental groups underlie some of the major conflicts that arise on any research project that tests the efficacy of a potentially beneficial intervention. In our case, the mandated standard intervention and the structure of the enhanced intervention, impact on all the components of the project from initial outreach to education and research and evaluation and differentially affect the project staff that are responsible for those components. In other words, there are many project requirements that are rooted in the research design but there are a large number of project staff who are not involved in the project as researchers; however, the requirements of the research impacts on their ability to do their job. The frequency with which operational issues arise gives us a barometer of how project requirements are working in the field. Over the past five years, staff from many project sites have talked a lot about the importance of ethnography in informing our data analyses; in a sense, almost each of our projects could also serve as an ethnographic case study of how things really work in the field.

The particular project functions and staff that we have in Philadelphia–but that are typical of other projects as well–include: (a) street outreach and project recruitment, which is performed by our community health educators or community health outreach workers (CHOWS); (b) interviewing, which is conducted by our interviewers; (c) HIV testing, counseling and standard intervention, which is the responsibility of our health educators; (d) enhanced intervention groups, conducted by health educators; and (e) research (designing the research, project management, data analysis, writing of reports/manuscripts, and proposal development). The research staff are engaged in these research activities with support from our data processing unit. Each of the staff have functions as defined within the parameters of the project and the conflicts that arise on a project like this often have their origin in the functions and protocols imposed on the staff. The staff sometimes operate under a set of conditions and circumstances which require them to respond somewhat differently than as mandated by the initial demands of the research design.

The definition that staff have of the project, as well as how they view the target population, impact on the daily balance between service and research. First, each type of staff person on the project has their own perspective or focus on what the project is about. As social scientists we know that the way things are defined often is a reflection of the world in which we operate and influences our behavior. As one would expect, the research staff see our project as a research project that involves a large service component. They are committed to the service component but they know that they have to maintain a level of scientific rigor to be able to assess whether or not our interventions are having an affect. Our analysis would be compromised if this level of control was not maintained. On the other hand, our service staff, primarily the CHOWS and Health Educators, really see this as an Acquired Immune Deficiency (AIDS) prevention project. They know that they are required to collect information because the project was funded by "the government."

The service staff adhere to collecting the information; however, in their day-to-day routine, the service staff talk to people on the street, talk to people in our field site office who often are desperate and at very high risk for HIV, as well as having numerous other health and social problems. As a consequence, the service staff are guided in their behavior and their values and beliefs by the clients with which they have to interact. Accordingly, the characteristics of our target population have an immediate impact on the ability of the outreach workers, the interviewers, and the health educators to follow the protocols and procedures. The target population is often times high, trying to deal with multiple personal crises, and is being asked to comply with requirements of being research subjects. It is significant that all the service staff refer to program participants as clients; they never talk about respondents or subjects. This reflects the fact that our service staff see our study participants within a clinical framework.

Differences in definitions of both the project and the target population impact on our ability to follow project protocols and require ongoing oversight and communication with service staff. These protocols involve: (a) record keeping; (b) sampling requirements; (c) information given in the standard intervention; (d) HIV testing; and (e) the structure of the enhanced intervention. What issues arise on a day-to-day basis? First, there is record keeping. There is a tremendous amount of data collection that takes place for all NADR and Cooperative Agreement sites. There are numerous steps in the project and at each step there are different data collection forms and information that needs to be gathered; these include: outreach, recruitment, field site operations, the consent form, urine samples, and verification of drug use, the Risk Behavior Assessment (RBA) and data trailer, information collected at first counseling session, information collected at the second counseling session, and information collected at a third (optional) counseling session. In addition, information is collected on persons who go through the enhanced intervention. Moreover, information is collected as we maintain follow-up contact with people and then, lastly, information collected at the time of the Risk Behavior Follow-Up Assessment (RBFA). Our field site is very hectic and much of the data are collected in this setting. As mentioned previously, the clients oftentimes come in a state of distress and all of this information has to be collected; the forms weigh over one-half pound. Collecting this information, which we do very well, involves an incredible balancing act and logistical precision.

Sampling is another area where there is often a need to review procedures and. adjust project service activities to comply with research requirements. The National Institute on Drug Abuse (NIDA) Cooperative Agreement sites have sampling quotas related to the kinds of people who must be recruited into the project. The primary sampling quota is based on type of drug use. Currently, projects are required to recruit 70% cocaine and 30% crack users. There are also quotas based on race and gender. These quotas may be different than what is found on the street and it always raises the issue of what is the appropriate target population? For example, in Philadelphia 55% of all persons who were admitted to treatment (in 1989) reported crack as their primary drug of abuse. This figure has probably increased; some information from the Philadelphia treatment system suggests it has. In one of the two neighborhoods in Philadelphia in which we work we have a distribution of Intravenous (IV) and crack users that is somewhat different from the assigned project quotas. In North Philadelphia, 70% of the drug users are IV users, 30% are crack users. In our second target neighborhood, in South Philadelphia, about 70% of the drug users are crack users and 30% are IV users. Accordingly, outreach workers will have to make many more contacts to secure the mandated sampling quotas in South Philadelphia.

In addition to record keeping and sampling requirements, there is always the need to balance the amount and type of information that can be and must be given out or communicated. Constraints on information may be contrary to the immediate needs of program clients and the situation in which staff find themselves. For example, outreach workers are not supposed to make any kind of active referrals. Our health educators are supposed to follow the protocols of the standard intervention in terms of the sequence of discussing the various information. But, as mentioned before, it is very difficult for outreach workers in our city, given our history as the NADR grantee and having a presence in the community, to simply serve as recruiters of study participants. Similarly, both outreach workers and health educators come into contact with clients or eligible respondents who are in a state of crisis and have an immediate problem with which both the client and our service staff have to deal. One of the health educators provided an apt example of such a situation: A woman had come into the field site office, she had just been interviewed and was distraught. It turns out that the client had been suffering physical abuse by her sexual partner and was extremely upset. The health educator felt that she could not go through the flash cards; she had to deal with the immediacy of the domestic violence situation. If fact, good clinical practice would probably be consistent with the way she approached this crisis. This is the type of situation the service staff confront daily. It's not that they fail to discuss the information on the flash cards, but it may be that at that moment those flash cards and the information that would be communicated would do more harm than good to the person sitting in front of you. However, in both of the above situations, we do collect information about whether referrals have been made and whether there was deviation from project protocols. In this manner, we can select out from future analyses those persons receiving "added" services or information.

As part of both the NADR and Cooperative Agreement Grant Programs project sites are required to collect data on the HIV status of program participants. In Philadelphia, HIV testing has always posed a dilemma. First, there is a paucity of services to which people can be referred; second, a large percentage of program participants have already been tested; and third, there is a great deal of denial and most clients who do get tested do not come back for their test results. All of these reasons have resulted in our health educators' deemphasizing HIV testing (the health educators are the ones who first introduce the subject of testing). We are trying to finally resolve this but, in Philadelphia at least, it has been an ongoing point of discussion for our project.[1] This issue illustrates the conflict between HIV testing that is offered as a service (with potential for referrals) versus HIV testing as epidemiologic data collection.

A final point with which the service and research staff have to deal involves the structure of the enhanced intervention. Philadelphia's enhanced intervention model was reconfigured between the NADR Program and Cooperative Agreement. This change was in response to the day-to-day realities of dealing with the target population. For example, when we first implemented the NADR project we did not really have experience, and neither did many of the other projects, in establishing interventions with the target population. In theory, we had a very nice structure outlined that involved a series of four cumulative education groups. The groups covered AIDS and risk factors associated with HIV, safer drug use, safer sex, and some special topics. The intervention model was structured so that each of these groups/topics met at a certain time on a certain day and people could come to the field site over a period of four weeks. Well, the lives of the target population are hectic and setting up such a structure was not workable. Now we have a more fluid, module

---

1. PHMC's Institutional Review Board has said that project staff may not offer any form of incentives related to HIV testing.

structure. Program participants can miss one topic and can go on to another topic because the current education sessions are not based on cumulative knowledge.

DISCUSSION

So what does this all mean in terms of running AIDS or other public health service projects that have a large research component or running research projects that have a large service component? Whether the issues discussed above arise and how they are resolved will, of course, depend on the way a project is defined, the needs of the city, community, and organization that is implementing the project and the resources that are available to offset the constraints imposed by research requirements. The above points are all related. Some of the things that we have done, or are trying to do in Philadelphia, include: (a) reorganizing the project management structure; (b) maximizing current resources; and (c) securing additional resources.

The Philadelphia NADR project was reorganized after the first year of operation to ensure greater sensitivity, coordination, and oversight of research and service components. When the project first began in Philadelphia in 1987, all project staff were housed within our Corporation's Research and Evaluation Division. The Principal Investigator was the key manager for the entire project. It became very clear over the first six months that the health educators, the outreach workers, and the referral coordinator had very different needs and different management requirements than those usually encountered by a research staff. It also became clear that the skills of the health educators and the outreach workers were transferrable across a broad range of projects in our Corporation; accordingly, the service staff was moved into a functional area that deals with health promotion and service systems. This reorganization resulted in a much more workable operational structure. This change did, however, place a requirement on the key research staff to engage in continuous communication with the managers of the service unit. This has been accomplished because of the interwoven nature of project components and also by regularly scheduled staff meetings. At these meetings emerging issues are discussed for the Cooperative Agreement program as well as for a number of our other AIDS-related projects.

Second, we responded to the research requirements and limited resources for service by altering our project design. In Philadelphia, we created a crossover design so as to maximize the outreach/ education resources that are available to the two target communities in which we work. In one of our target communities (North Philadelphia) all persons are eligible for the enhanced intervention and in our second community (South Philadelphia), persons are currently eligible for just the standard intervention. In eighteen months, we will reverse this eligibility.

Finally, we have also tried to respond to the limited service resources by securing additional funding from local, state, and other federal agencies. Of course, when you attempt to get additional funding it is crucial to secure these funds in a timely fashion and for a purpose which is consistent with the goals of the existing project. There are many requests for proposals that get issued and some of them will fund outreach workers and some of them will fund health educators. Oftentimes these programs have unique foci and purposes. The latter is particularly relevant when responding to federal program announcements. Some new projects cannot be easily integrated or coordinated with an existing program. Therefore, it may be difficult to rely upon federal agencies for additional sources of funds. Accordingly, it will be necessary to secure local and state funding for ongoing service activities. It is important to continue these projects not only beyond NADR but beyond the Cooperative Agreement program, as well.

In sum, the need to strike a balance between the demands of prevention research and service will always exist for programs that are attempting to undertake both types of activities. The ability to understand areas of conflict and derive solutions is all the more crucial in AIDS research and service demonstration programs. As an original NADR site, Philadelphia project staff–as well as staff in other cities–felt like they were going through a rite of passage; some of us said, "We will never do this again!" In point of fact, when the Cooperative Agreement proposal request was released, we looked at it and we said, "Well, we have to do this again. People are dying, there is an epidemic, and we seem to be making some impact on our communities." The progress that has been made to date, and the commitment it has engendered, will require us to continue to balance the need for service in our community with the need to collect information which is scientifically rigorous. At the same time, there is a growing need to fund services that will continue and/or expand upon those models which have proven to be successful. In a sense, this is the ultimate challenge faced by persons engaged in prevention/intervention research.

The Significance of Sampling and Understanding Hidden Populations

John K. Watters, PhD

SUMMARY. Discussed are issues related to the importance of sampling from hidden populations in research. These issues include the limitations of dependency on institutional samples in public health and social science. Specific examples are drawn from research into HIV/AIDS infection and risk behaviors and substance abuse. Discussed is the problem of developing knowledge that does not generalize to non-institutional populations. Possible future directions for research in hidden populations in the context of HIV/AIDS research are addressed.

INTRODUCTION

It is axiomatic that there is frequently tension between what is *feasible* and what is *desirable*. In the social sciences, epidemiology,

John K. Watters is Associate Professor, School of Medicine, University of California, San Francisco with joint appointments in the Department of Family and Community Medicine, and the Institute for Health Policy Studies.

The author gratefully acknowledges the support of the Center for Alcohol and Addiction Studies, University of Alaska Anchorage; the National Institute on Drug Abuse (grant # U01 DA 06908); and the AIDS Office of the San Francisco Department of Public Health.

Correspondence may be addressed to the author at: School of Medicine, Box 1304, University of California, San Francisco, CA 94143-1304.

An earlier version of this paper was presented at the "AIDS Prevention Symposium," University of Alaska Anchorage, May 6, 1992.

[Haworth co-indexing entry note]: "The Significance of Sampling and Understanding Hidden Populations." Watters, John K. Co-published simultaneously in *Drugs & Society* (The Haworth Press, Inc.) Vol. 7, No. 3/4, 1993, pp. 13-21; and: *AIDS and Community-Based Drug Intervention Programs: Evaluation and Outreach* (ed: Dennis G. Fisher, and Richard Needle) The Haworth Press, Inc., 1993, pp. 13-21. Multiple copies of this article/chapter may be purchased from The Haworth Document Delivery Center [1-800-3-HAWORTH; 9:00 a.m. - 5:00 p.m. (EST)].

Copyright © 1993 by Taylor & Francis

and public health this tension is considerable. The great preponderance of scientific knowledge about various social and psychological phenomena of interest to these overlapping fields of inquiry is the result of institutionally-based research. Some examples are intelligence (from public schools), crime and delinquency (from correctional settings and courts), and psychological states and traits (from college undergraduates). There is a long and illustrious intellectual tradition in the study of institutional populations in psychology, the sociology of deviance, and substance abuse. In many instances, such studies are extremely valuable. They provide a basis for understanding characteristics of common populations. Such studies are limited because findings derived from institutional populations may not generalize to their non-institutional counterparts. Non-institutional populations may differ in terms of various key attributes such as experience, education, ethnicity, motivation, beliefs, attitudes, values, goals and economics, to name but a few.

Some investigators have attempted to control for this source of bias by generating probability samples. Of course, the problem with this strategy is that "hidden populations" such as homeless persons and drug injectors rarely appear in such surveys. Consequently, the U.S. Census Bureau, in a major shift in traditional practices, has instituted an attempt to "enumerate" homeless persons.

The national "Monitoring the Future Study" (high school senior survey) has queried seniors in a national panel of high schools about their drug and alcohol use (National Institute of Drug Abuse [NIDA], 1987). These data are used for various purposes, both scientific and political, and have been used to derive estimates of the relative success of federal drug prevention efforts. The problem here is that youth who drop out of school before the survey is taken (during their senior year) remain hidden from this national surveillance. One might argue that those who do drop out are at elevated risk for participation in drug use relative to those who succeed in making it into their senior year of high school. So, while the "Senior Survey" is an enormously useful data source, it is limited in that it relies completely on an institutional population that we may assume differ in terms of key characteristics from their hidden counterparts–high school drop-outs. While it is desirable to survey drop-outs, the feasibility of this approach poses many methodological, logistical, and economic challenges to those interested in the changing epidemiology of substance use among youth.

Another probability sample that attempts to determine levels of drug and alcohol consumption is the "National Household Survey." The results of this survey are significant and provide useful data (NIDA, 1989, 1990). Unfortunately, this design is limited because like the survey of high-school seniors, it fails to canvas persons who are outside of stable domiciles. This population may be at greater risk for problems associated with alcohol and drug use than those with relatively permanent addresses. Despite the limitation of these sampling strategies, and in the absence of data about hidden populations, data from these surveys serves as the scientific foundation for many health policy decisions regarding substance abuse (U.S. Public Health Service [PHS], 1991).

SAMPLING IN HIDDEN POPULATIONS

Much of what we accept as knowledge about drug users has been based upon research with drug treatment program clients, and most frequently clients enrolled in some form of methadone-based treatment. This has begun to change in recent years, with several important research initiatives now sponsored in the United States by the Centers for Disease Control (CDC) and The National Institute on Drug Abuse (NIDA). These initiatives specifically target hidden populations of injection drug users and/or crack cocaine users in their natural environments. These studies represent a major departure from traditional substance abuse research. They combine quantitative and qualitative methodologies to begin to understand a cluster of health policy related issues relevant to this population. The primary impetus behind this fledgling research agenda has been concern over rising AIDS cases in drug users. Nevertheless, the methods used and knowledge developed in the course of these projects has significance beyond the AIDS epidemic, and represent the first large scale efforts to systematically study non-institutional populations of drug users.

Some of the CDC and NIDA efforts employ some form of research strategies that are loosely based upon or derived from "targeted sampling" (Watters & Biernacki, 1989). Briefly, targeted sampling is a collection of research methods or strategies that generate sufficient numbers of members of hidden populations for systematic, quantitative study. Samples are developed by first defining the characteristics of interest (say, injection drug users not enrolled in drug treatment programs). Then, through a series of steps, methods are established that permit systematic recruiting of samples of the targeted population. As such, targeted sampling draws heavily on elements of ethnography, survey sampling, theoretical sampling, and snowball sampling. It is not a method for generating random samples, and there is considerable room for sampling error for this reason. Targeted sampling is not intended to be a rigid framework for conducting research among hidden populations, but rather provides some flexible guidelines and principles for generating non-institutional samples.

Targeting Hidden Populations in the Context of HIV/AIDS Research and Intervention

Why are these developments important? The most compelling reason is that we cannot estimate either the current or future size of the Human Immunodeficiency Virus (HIV) epidemic without a better understanding of the size and composition of the drug using population. For example, in the United States, the primary means of HIV surveillance for drug users is the CDC Family of Surveys. This enormously useful mechanism recruits volunteers in methadone treatment clinics in selected metropolitan areas for HIV testing. Leaving aside the question of non-injecting drug users (e.g., crack cocaine smokers), this means of surveillance samples exclusively within the estimated 15% of injection drug users (IDUs) who are enrolled in drug treatment (Wiley & Samuel, 1989). The vast majority of IDUs remain completely outside of the surveillance system. The CDC Family of Surveys accrues significant bias through total dependence on its institutional samples because the system excludes those individuals who are not eligible for methadone treatment due to their primary reliance on injected drugs other than opiates (e.g., cocaine and/or amphetamines), because they are not "daily" injectors, because they cannot successfully complete the long waiting period that is typically associated with entry into treatment, because they are otherwise unmotivated to enter treatment, or because they live in geographical areas that are remote from treatment units included in the Family of Surveys panel.

A less biased survey that provides a means for estimating the size and composition of the HIV epidemic among IUDs exists in the CDC AIDS case data. From these data one can discern that heterosexual IDUs represent the second leading (and fastest growing) risk category for AIDS in the U.S. (23% during 1991; CDC, 1992), and that these cases are disproportionately African American and Hispanic. These data also suggest that over half of the pediatric cases of AIDS have resulted from at least one parent's involvement with injected drugs or an infected injection drug user. These data are terribly important, but as a means for directing prevention efforts and identifying recent outbreaks of HIV infection they are seriously limited for two reasons. First, an AIDS diagnosis is a relatively late development in the HIV disease process. In most cases, actual infection would have occurred years prior to diagnosis. Consequently, AIDS case data provide a glimpse of where the rising tide of infection was years prior to the actual year of diagnosis of disease. Second, the term "AIDS" is a CDC-generated case definition. To obtain an AIDS diagnosis, in addition to confirmation of HIV infection, a specific set of clinical criteria must be met. This means that many individuals may die of infections that are secondary to their weakened immune system that are not "AIDS definition" disease (Stoneburner, Des Jarlais, Benezara et al., 1988). Since these cases of HIV-related mortality will not carry the CDC case definition, AIDS case data may seriously underestimate the true size of the epidemic (Andrulis, Weslowski, Hintz, & Spolarich, 1992).

THE APPEARANCE OF ELEPHANTS TO THE BLIND

The story of the blind men who seek to know what an elephant is like may be a useful metaphor for what we know about HIV epidemics. In this parable, each blind man described the elephant differently. For each, the beast was like the part he had examined with his outstretched hands. For each the experience and the conclusion were different. One had felt the animal's leg, another its broad side, still another the tail, and so on. Each had different knowledge based on their different observation, and each was convinced of the veracity of his conclusions. This is not unlike HIV epidemics, where the features that we see are those that are illuminated by AIDS case data, the findings of the CDC Family of Surveys, and the patchwork of seroprevalence data that emerges from other studies. The vast majority of these sources are institutional data, and as a result, we still have a very limited view of non-institutional populations. This may be especially true of IDUs. For all of these reasons, there exist many problem areas in the capacity of current surveillance efforts to project future cases, locate emerging outbreaks, and target intervention efforts where they will have the greatest effect. Consequently, while a great deal is known about the size, composition, and direction of the HIV/AIDS epidemic, our incomplete picture looks something like an elephant to a blind man. The conclusions we draw about the HIV/AIDS epidemics depends upon which general part of the elephant we grope with our outstretched hands.

One illustration of this problem can be seen when the results of targeted samples of IDUs are compared with institutional samples. In an earlier study, IDUs in San Francisco who were enrolled in drug treatment were less likely to be infected with HIV than those out-of-treatment (Watters & Cheng, 1987). In a more recent study in the San Francisco Bay Area, HIV rates derived from targeted samples were compared with those obtained from the CDC Family of Surveys for three Bay Area counties (Watters, 1992). In each instance, the targeted samples showed higher rates of HIV seroprevalence rates than were reflected in the in-treatment population. These differences ranged from a factor of 1.7 to 2.1 higher in the targeted samples. In one of these counties the HIV seroprevalence rate reported for IDUs by the Family of Surveys has consistently been about 5%. However, in one predominately African American community in this county, an infection rate of 18% was found–about four times that of the county level data obtained from the Family of Surveys. Consequently, the conclusions we draw about the size and composition of HIV epidemics may be profoundly influenced by choice of sampling method and the locations chosen to sample. This leaves those of us who are determined to understand the dimensions of HIV (or other) epidemics with problems not unlike those that confronted the blind men who examined the elephant.

SOME POSSIBLE FUTURE DIRECTIONS

While targeted sampling can provide useful access to and new knowledge about segments of society that are rarely viewed, there remain many pitfalls in the application of this set of techniques in the context of the HIV/AIDS epidemic. For example, sampling of hidden populations for seroprevalence and/or seroincidence studies could be strengthened if developed systematically, not just at the local or regional level, but at the national level as well. Failure to accomplish this will inhibit studies of non-institutional populations from meeting their full potential. For example, the current array of surveillance data could be significantly enhanced with a national program of targeted samples in selected metropolitan and non-metropolitan areas throughout the United States. Current efforts do have some capacity to illuminate specific risk practices and HIV infection rates in the few communities where established. However, these efforts do not provide a consistent panel of reporting sites selected on explicit criteria relevant to tracking HIV infection, changes in drug use practices, or levels of sexual risk. Such a national sample could be developed by targeting communities that meet specific criteria in terms of demographics and other indicators using strategies incorporated in targeted sampling but applied on a larger scale. Such an approach would seem to be highly desirable because of its ability to provide information on the leading indicators of epidemic outbreaks (infection rates) and behavioral risks as well as drug abuse epidemiology prior to the fact of disease diagnosis. Although it would seem to be desirable, an effort of this type may not, however, be feasible, based on the availability of funding, qualified researchers, and the overall climate of receptiveness to non-institutional studies. The current portfolio of studies of hidden populations does include a number of major metropolitan areas and smaller communities, the coverage is spotty at best, and, in some ways, represents a "convenience sample" of locations for study that is based more on the vagaries of grant and contract competition than on a systematic effort to sample communities at risk. The same can be said of intervention efforts directed at the risk populations of IDUs and their sexual partners.

Nevertheless, despite these limitations, the emergence of large scale studies of hidden populations is a significant step forward. We have the opportunity to acquire significant new knowledge, and use these projects as vehicles for applying this knowledge to disease intervention efforts that can be systematically evaluated to determine their efficacy. There is some evidence emerging from NIDA's National AIDS Demonstration Research effort that the fundamental research enterprize of HIV testing and counseling, accomplished in conjunction with a thorough individualized risk assessment may represent a significant prevention effort in its own right (Stevens & Simpson, 1992). Such efforts are often a primary source of HIV/AIDS prevention messages driven home by the medical fact of the antibody test result when delivered. This combination of laborious recall of risk history coupled with the HIV antibody test can be a powerful means for HIV/AIDS education among a very high risk population.

In addition to their prevention value, these efforts can serve a useful case-finding mechanism for referral to HIV disease treatment and intervention with sexual partners. While treatment of HIV infected individuals is still in its infancy, there are more weapons in the physicians' armamentarium than at the outset of the epidemic. Antiviral therapies (such as AZT) may extend life. Other preventative measures include the use of aerosolized pentamidine for the prevention of *Pneumocystis carinii* pneumonia (common among HIV infected IDUs; CDC, 1992b), and revised protocols for the treatment of infection with *Mycobacterium tuberculosis* in individuals co-infected with HIV (a growing epidemic among IDUs; CDC, 1990; Selwyn et al., 1989).

REFERENCES

Andrulis, D.P., Weslowski, V.B., Hintz, E., & Spolarich, A.W. (1992). Comparisons of hospital care for patients with AIDS and other HIV related conditions. *Journal of the American Medical Association, 267,* 2482-2486.
Centers for Disease Control. (1990). Screening for tuberculosis infection in high-

risk populations, and the use of preventive therapy for tuberculosis infection in the United States: Recommendations of the advisory committee for elimination of tuberculosis. *Morbidity and Mortality Weekly Review, 39*, 1-12.

Centers for Disease Control. (1992). *HIV/AIDS Surveillance: First quarter edition. U.S. AIDS cases reported through March 1992.* Atlanta, GA: U.S. Dept. of Health and Human Services, Centers for Disease Control, National Center for Infectious Diseases, Division of HIV/AIDS.

Centers for Disease Control. (1992b). Recommendations for prophylaxis against *Pneumocystis carinii* pneumonia for adults and adolescents infected with HIV. *Morbidity and Mortality Weekly Review, 41*, 1-12.

National Institute on Drug Abuse. (1987). *National trends in drug use and related factors among American high school students and young adults, 1975-1986.* DHHS Pub. No. (ADM)87-1535. Washington, DC: U.S. Department of Health and Human Services.

National Institute on Drug Abuse. (1989). *Household survey on drug abuse: Population estimates 1988*: DHHS Pub. No. (ADM)90-1682. Washington, DC: U.S. Department of Health and Human Services.

Selwyn, P.A., Hartell, D., Lewis, V.A., Schoenbaum, E.E., Sten, H.V., Klein, R.S., Walker, A.T., & Friedland, G.H. (1989). A prospective study of the risk of tuberculosis among intravenous drug users with human immunodeficiency virus infection. *The New England Journal of Medicine, 320*, 545-549.

Stevens, R., & Simpson D. (1992, May). *NADR project experiences: "What have we learned?"* Presentation at NIDA Cooperative Agreement Steering Committee Meeting, Anchorage, AK.

Stoneburner, R.L., Des Jarlais, D.C., Benezara, D. et al. (1988). A larger spectrum of HIV severe HIV-1-related disease in intravenous drug users in New York City. *Science, 242*, 916-919.

U.S. Public Health Service. (1991). *Healthy people 2000: National health promotion and disease prevention objectives.* DHHS Pub. No. (PHS)91-50212. Washington, DC: U.S. Department of Health and Human Services.

Watters, J.K., & Biernacki, P. (1989). Targeted sampling: Options for the study of hidden populations. *Social Problems, 36*, 416-430.

Watters, J.K., & Cheng, Y-T. (1987). HIV infection and risk among intravenous drug users in San Francisco: Preliminary findings. *Contemporary Drug Problems, 14*, 397-410.

Watters, J.K. (1992, May). The epidemiology of HIV in Drug Injectors in the San Francisco Bay Area. Paper presented at the AIDS Prevention Symposium, Anchorage, AK.

Wiley, J.A., & Samuel, M.C. (1989). Prevalence of HIV infection in the USA. *AIDS, 3* (supplement 1), S71-S78.

Pile Sorts, A Cognitive Anthropological Model of Drug and AIDS Risks for Navajo Teenagers: Assessment of a New Evaluation Tool

Robert T. Trotter II, PhD
James M. Potter, BA

SUMMARY. This article presents data which support the use of a cognitive anthropology research method, "pile sorting," to compliment and enhance the qualitative and quantitative evaluation tools used by drug prevention programs. The method was employed in the assessment of a Drug, Alcohol, and AIDS prevention program conducted by a community based organization. It produced significant information on the cognitive models of risks held by Native American teenagers, and provided a method of determining target areas for revision of the prevention and intervention program, as well as

Robert T. Trotter II is Professor and Chair, Department of Anthropology, Northern Arizona University. James M. Potter is a graduate student, Department of Anthropology and is Outreach Coordinator for the Flagstaff Multi-Cultural Aids Prevention Project.

Mailing address: Department of Anthropology, Campus Box 15200, Northern Arizona University, Flagstaff, AZ 86011.

The analysis of the data presented was supported by NIDA Grant # U01 DA07295-01, from the National Institute on Drug Abuse.

[Haworth co-indexing entry note]: "Pile Sorts, A Cognitive Anthropological Model of Drug and AIDS Risks for Navajo Teenagers: Assessment of a New Evaluation Tool." Trotter, Robert T. II, and James M. Potter. Co-published simultaneously in *Drugs & Society* (The Haworth Press, Inc.) Vol. 7, No. 3/4, 1993, pp. 23-39; and: *AIDS and Community-Based Drug Intervention Programs: Evaluation and Outreach* (ed: Dennis G. Fisher, and Richard Needle) The Haworth Press, Inc., 1993, pp. 23-39. Multiple copies of this article/chapter may be purchased from The Haworth Document Delivery Center [1-800-3-HAWORTH; 9:00 a.m. - 5:00 p.m. (EST)].

Copyright © 1993 by Taylor & Francis

assessing the impact of the existing program. Pile sorting proved to be simple to administer, fun for respondents, and provided analytical information at a positive ratio between time-on-task compared to richness of result.

INTRODUCTION

This paper explores the potential for using a cognitive anthropology method, called "pile sorting" (Weller and Romney 1988) to evaluate drug and HIV risk prevention programs. The technique was developed to assess culturally defined taxonomic relationships (Roberts et al. 1980) and has subsequently proven extremely useful in accurate cognitive mapping of ecological issues. Boster and Johnson (1989) demonstrated an effective use of pile sorts to establish models of the underlying cultural relationships between species of fish which are favored or avoided by sports fishermen in the United States. This led to successful efforts to reduce ecological pressure on over-fished species, and an increased utilization of under-fished species on the Florida coast. Their achievement raises the possibility of applying the method to other areas of prevention and intervention.

We hypothesized that analyzing a group's cultural depiction of the relationships among drug, alcohol, HIV and other risks might lead to practical uses for this technique. Therefore the authors conducted a study to determine whether pile sorting could assist the evaluation of a program to reduce behaviors which place Native American teenagers at risk through drug use, sexual encounters, school drop-out and other problems.

BACKGROUND FOR THE STUDY

Navajo and other Native American teenagers are at high risk for drug and alcohol related conditions, school problems, car accidents, and family disruption (Lamarine 1988, Beauvais et al. 1989). They are at increasing risk from HIV infection (Metler et al. 1991, Blum et al. 1992), as indicated by key co-morbidity markers for HIV, such as sexually transmitted diseases (Toomey et al. 1989). Efforts have been undertaken by tribal officials, local community groups and others to increase Native American teenagers' awareness of the risks of drug abuse, HIV infection, and other problems. These efforts include media campaigns, health fairs, and in-school AIDS awareness and prevention projects (Rolf et al. 1991a). The result is an increasing awareness of the most common drug and alcohol problems as well as the standard modes of transmission of the HIV virus, in terms of unprotected sexual contact and needle sharing among drug users (Rolf et al, 1991a, 1991b).

METHODOLOGICAL AND THEORETICAL CONSIDERATIONS

The pile sort technique produces unconstrained clusters of the items being sorted. These clusters are representative of a cultural taxonomy, which can then be transformed into individual and composite distance matrices using available computer programs such as ANTHROPAC.[1] The aggregate matrix produces an averaged group view of the relationships among these variables. There are two standard ways of analyzing and presenting this data; through the use of cluster analysis, and through multidimensional scaling. Both produce visual and quantitative representations of the data, which can be analyzed by the researcher solely as a test of a hypothesis, or can be returned for further exploration and commentary by informants, or both.

We initiated a base line standard for our project that the pile sort method meet the following criteria, in order to demonstrate its effectiveness as an evaluation tool. The first condition is that the technique provide us data that clearly recapitulates data derived by other methodological approaches, thus providing a measure of the validity of the method by demanding that pile sorts show the same relationships that can be found within original open ended ethnographic or quantitative interview data collected on the target cultural domain. The pile sort analysis should exhibit the same type and direction of linkages and interactions between the risks that would be found by other research methods. The second standard is that the technique should be capable of showing a change in relationships that reflects a change in the way that our respondents think and talk about the risks. If these base line conditions are supported by the analysis of the pile sort data, we feel that we can demonstrate a practical drug program application for this technique.

METHODOLOGY

In 1992 a group of Native American teenagers received an AIDS, drug, and alcohol risk prevention program sponsored by a local community organization, NACA,[2] in Flagstaff, Arizona. The primary goal for the NACA intervention was to offer education about choices pertaining to alcohol, drugs, sex relations, IV drug use, and their relationship to AIDS. Considerable time was spent dealing with alcohol use and drug use related to family problems. Avenues of HIV transmission were discussed and special emphasis was placed on sexual activity and the use of condoms, but only limited information was presented on the relationship between injection drug use and HIV transmission. This program provided an opportunity to pilot test the pile sort evaluation technique.

Based on previous research on the Navajo Reservation (Trotter et al., in press), we created a set of variables that described the cultural domain of risk taking for Native American teenagers, sub-divided by risk clusters. The categories and the individual risks selected for exploration in our pile sort research were then chosen by a panel composed of Navajo and non-Native American project personnel, following extensive ethnographic work. Those categories are listed below, as they were printed on the pile sort stimulus cards. The letters associated with each risk (used as identifiers in the cluster analysis and multidimensional scaling plots) result from a randomization of all of the risk factors, to avoid the bias of placing the original risk clusters together during their presentation to the respondents.

1. Drug Related Risks

The focus group discussions of drug risks included the drugs available on and off the reservation, descriptions of the types of behaviors that were engaged in by people who use drugs, the risks associated with drug use (including harm to self and harm to others). The panel included the following risks from this set: *C.* Using More Than One Drug at the Same Time; *E.* Sniffing Something to Get High; *R.* Getting High; *X.* Marijuana; *Z.* Using IV Drugs (Needle Drugs); *g.* Smoking Cigarettes.

2. Alcohol Related Risks

The Navajo teenager and adult interviews explored the alcoholic beverages available on and off the reservation, descriptions of the behaviors of people who drink, and the risks associated with drinking (including harm to self and harm to others). The risk cards contain the following items: *H.* Drinking Hard Liquor (Whisky, Vodka, Gin, Tequila, Etc.); *K.* Drinking; *L.* Cruising Around in a Car and Drinking; *P.* Passing Out; *a.* Drinking Wine; *h.* You Can't Remember What Happened While You Were High or Drunk; *i.* Someone Getting You Drunk When You Don't Want To; *o.* Drinking Beer.

3. Sexual and HIV Related Risks

Our ethnographic interviews determined what our respondents knew about sex and the causes of HIV infection, how it could be reduced through protective practices, how concerned they were about AIDS, and what they thought could be done to reduce the risk of HIV infection on and off the reservation. The risk factors presented to the respondents included: *A.* Unprotected Sex; *B.* Having Sex Frequently; *G.* Having Lots of Sex Partners; *I.* Raping Someone; *Q.* AIDS; *S.* Having Sex without Birth Control; *T.* Getting Pregnant; *U.* Venereal Diseases (STD's); *W.* Getting Someone Pregnant; *k.* Having Unwanted Sex or Intercourse; *n.* Getting Raped; *p.* Having Sex with Someone You Don't Know.

4. School Related Risks

School risk discussions included academic risk (poor grades and dropping out) as well as problems in peer relationships and relationships with teachers and parents that were connected to school. The risks chosen for inclusion included: *J.* Poor Grades or Flunking Out of School; *O.* Dropping Out of School; *V.* Ditching School; *f.* Doing Something that Gets You Suspended from School; *l.* Not Doing Your Homework; *m.* Showing Disrespect for Parents or Teachers.

5. Family Violence and Personal Violence Risks

The risks mentioned about family relationships included family violence, alcohol and drug abuse, and school pressures. The other violence related risks included dares, hazardous driving, suicide, fights with others, and other forms of interpersonal conflict. Some of these risks were placed in other categories, based on primarily associations during the discussions. The remaining family or individual risks (from interpersonal conflict, dares, or accidents) were placed in this category: *D.* Hurting Yourself; *F.* Family Violence; *M.* Driving Fast; *N.* Riding With Someone Who is Driving Dangerously; *Y.* Beating Someone Up; *c.* Getting in Fights; *d.* Harassing People; *e.* Suicide Attempts; *q.* Car Accidents.

6. Two Risks from Traditional Beliefs

Only 41 of the 43 risks presented to the students come from the original ethnographic data sets. At the suggestion of one of the panel members, two risks from Navajo traditional beliefs were added as comparative spiritual or supernatural markers for these physical and social risks. The traditional risks are: *b.* Walking Around in a Lightning Storm and *j.* Walking Home Alone at Night.

The 43 risks were presented on individual cards, with the letter designator for the risk on the back to assist in data recording. The sorts were accomplished by laying the risk cards out in identically ordered rows in front of each respondent, so they could see all of the risks at the same time. We asked the students to look at the risks and then place them in piles, according to the ones that they felt go together. They were told they could make as many or as few piles as they wanted, and could put the cards together on the basis of anything that they think appropriate. The data were recorded by noting the individual risks placed in each pile by each respondent, as well as the total number of piles created. We also recorded the answer to the question, "why did you put these things in this pile," for each of the respondent's piles.

The data reported in this article were collected from Navajo males ranging in age from 18 to 19 years old. The pretest data set was collected from 11 students prior to their taking the NACA Drugs, Alcohol, and AIDS awareness program. The posttest set was collected from 17 students who completed the NACA program. Six students completed both the pretest and the posttest, the others completed only one of the two tasks. Since this pilot study was designed as a preliminary methodological test of the processes, rather than an attempt to thoroughly explore all of the interconnections of risks for these groups, it was felt that this collected sufficiently reliable data to either recommend the technique be employed in larger projects, or suggest that the technique was not worth pursuing on a larger scale, according to suggested sample sizes for this type of task (Kruskal and Wish 1978). The results from the pilot are also very consistent with the results from pile sorts we ran on comparable (but larger) groups (Trotter, Potter, Price 1993), which enhances our confidence in the technique.

DATA AND ANALYSIS

Pile sort distance matrices produced by ANTHROPAC were analyzed using cluster analysis and multidimensional scaling to demonstrate either the hierarchical relationships of the risks to one another, or the latent structure inherent in the relationships of the variables to one another in multidimensional space.

The following dendrogram depicts the hierarchical cluster relationships as they were created by the Native American teenagers during the pretest pile sort data collection (Figure 1).

The data support two of the relational considerations discussed in the theory section. The basic clusters of risks that were identified by the panel members, from the ethnographic data, have been recapitulated by the pile sort technique, even though the risks were randomized. Reading from the left of the dendrogram, the first six elements are school risks ("O" through "m"), the following 13 ("Q"

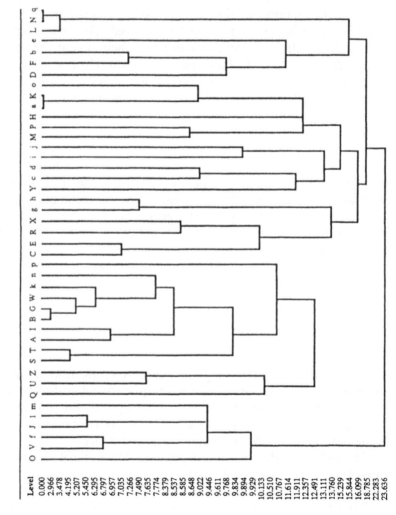

FIGURE 1. Pre-test Cluster Analysis

through "p") are the sex and HIV risks, with the exception of "Z," which is IV Drugs (Needle Drugs). The subsequent set "C" through "g" are the drug cluster. The placement of "Z," IV Drugs, indicates that some of the students were associating HIV and IV Drug risks at this level or relationship.

This dendrogram indicates significant inter-relationships between the family and individual violence risks and the alcohol related risks (the variables "h" through "q" in the dendrogram). This configuration was similar to that found in the ethnographic data which preceded the project. Some of the risks interconnect at close or strong levels, such as "N" and "q" (riding with someone who is driving dangerously and car accidents), while others remain more cognitively separated in their relationship, as with "n" and "p" (getting raped and having sex with someone you don't know).

The cluster analysis performed on the posttest data allowed us to generate a time-two analysis of the data (Figure 2).

This dendrogram presents the relationships among risks for the posttest which shows some key differences compared with the first analysis. Most of the clusters are stable, and in some instances have been strengthened. For example, beginning at the left of the dendrogram, "Q" through "p" are the sex and HIV risks. This time, IV Drugs is embedded in the drug cluster ("C" through "Z"), and the cigarettes variable has moved into the alcohol related risks. This indicates that the underlying domain structure, and the boundaries between domains, were strengthened by the intervention (or external education), since some interconnections were reformulated. Strengthening these associations was one of the goals of the intervention, and this outcome indicates success in this attempt. As with the first dendrogram, the strongest cross-group associations are between alcohol related risks and family and personal violence related risks.

The dendrograms have a limited utility for exploring the highly complex latent structural relationships captured in the pile sort data. Therefore, we conducted a second analysis of the data using multi-dimensional scaling. The MDS data creates visual depictions for all of the n dimensional combinations of the variables. We analyzed the statistical and graphic summaries of 4 dimensions in this data set: 1 by 2, 1 by 3, 1 by 4, 2 by 3, 2 by 4 and 3 by 4. Only the representa-

FIGURE 2. Post-test Cluster Analysis

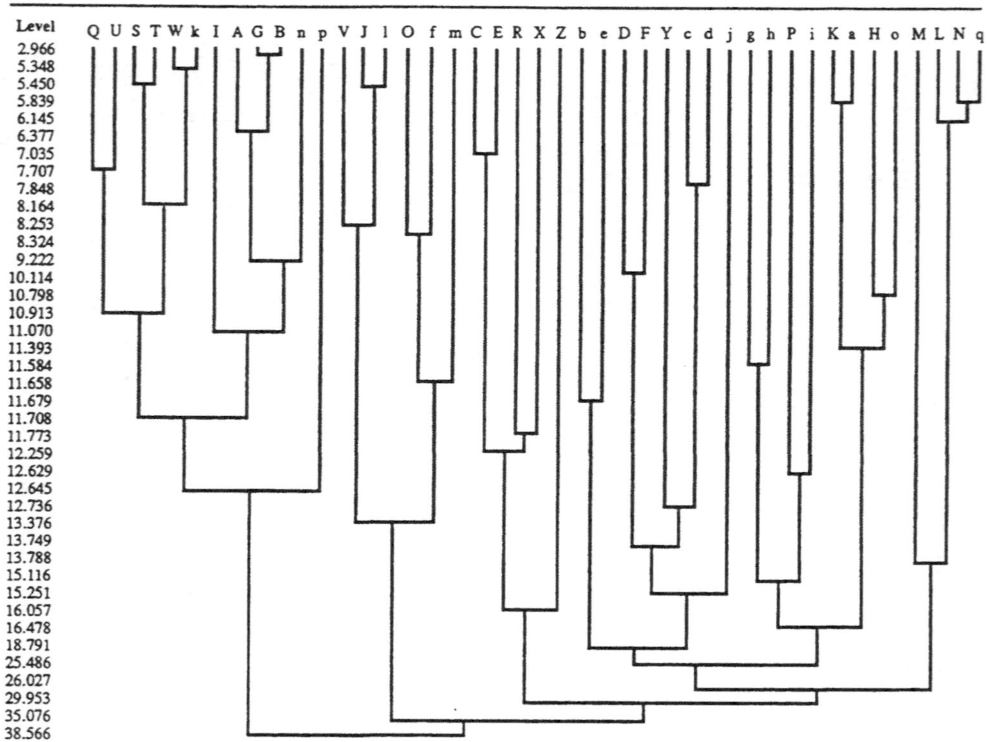

tions of two of these dimensional comparisons are presented below, due to space limitations. The other plots show similar relationships between the sex and the drug variables, which are the focus of this paper, although they indicate differences among the other risk clusters, which would be worthy of further exploration for a different forum.

Two pretest MDS plots were chosen to show the maximum demarcation of the original, panel created, risk domains (Figure 3), and the maximum integration of these multiple domains (Figure 4).

In evaluating the preceding two plots, note the separation of the HIV

FIGURE 3. Pretest MDS Plot 1

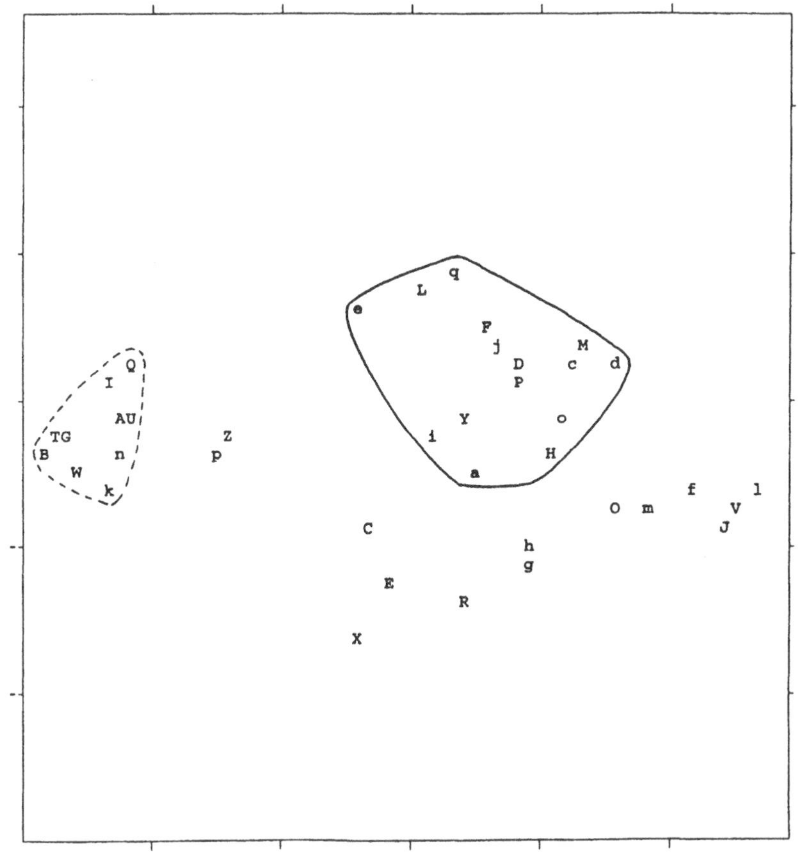

FIGURE 4. Pretest MDS Plot 2

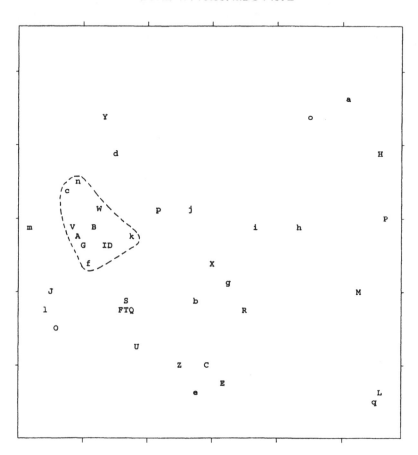

and sexual risk constellation (the letters inside the dotted line) from other risks in Figure 3, while there is clear interpenetration of alcohol, family violence, and individual violence risks (indicated by letters enclosed by solid line in Figure 3). The drug risks and school risks also form distinct, non-interrelated clusters. Only one relationship is depicted between IV drugs and a sex risk, in this case "p," having sex with someone you don't know. These data support the conditions presented in the introduction, in relation to recapitulating the ethnographic data. The students have recreated most of the original domains we derived from the qualitative interview data, in both the cluster analysis and the MDS data above, even when using randomized stimuli.

Pretest plot 2 provides a different dimensional view of the data. In this case, the dimensions chosen for display provide the greatest degree of interpenetration and multiple relationships between the risks. The risk variables enclosed in the dotted lines (Figure 4) come from three risk clusters, sex related risks, school risks, and family and personal violence. This cluster depicts close connections between ditching school ("V") and two sex risks, unprotected sex ("A"), and having lots of sex partners ("G"), as an example. In other clusters there are relationships between drug risks and violence risks, and alcohol and violence risks, all of which are associations between these risks that were embedded in the original ethnographic data collected to define the risks to the students.

Following the NACA AIDS intervention program, we conducted a posttest using the same risk cards and instructions used in the pretest. The following two MDS plots offer a visual representation of the results.

The posttest MDS plots again support the theoretical and practical considerations for this paper. One of the most important findings is that an intervention can build stronger relationships within the risk clusters, at the expense of inter-cluster relationships. The NACA intervention was designed to reinforce the importance of the relationship between unprotected sex and AIDS, and spent far less time showing interrelationships between IV Drugs and AIDS, with the consequence that the IVDU-HIV interconnections at posttest are more tenuous than at pretest, while the sex and alcohol risk domains have been strongly reinforced. There are fewer interrelationships between alcohol and violence risks, in the posttest MDS plots, but more between sex and drugs, which is complimentary to the expected outcome of the intervention. Figure 5 again shows the original clusters, tightened in space by the reinforcement of the NACA intervention. For comparison with the other figures, the sex risks are on the left hand side of the plot, enclosed in dotted lines. The strongest area of integration of variables, enclosed in a solid line, includes the inter-relationships of alcohol, drug, and drunk driving risks.

FIGURE 5. Post-test MDS Plot 1

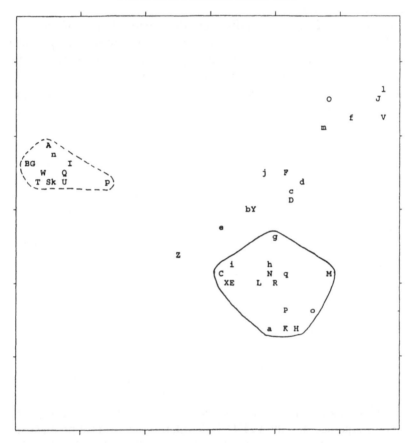

The posttest MDS data confirms the increased distance between IV Drugs and both AIDS and STD's along all dimensions except the one depicted in Figure 6, where there is a relatively weak relationship visible within the cluster of variables enclosed in the dotted line. Figure 6 also depicts the success of the NACA intervention by showing the students relate sexual risks to other areas of their lives, and in particular alcohol and school problems. For example, having unwanted sex "k" is related to not being able to remember what happened when you were high "h" and to getting raped "n." IV Drugs "Z" are related to dropping out of school "O" and not doing your homework "L." Thus, there is an indication that some new

FIGURE 6. Post-test MDS Plot 2

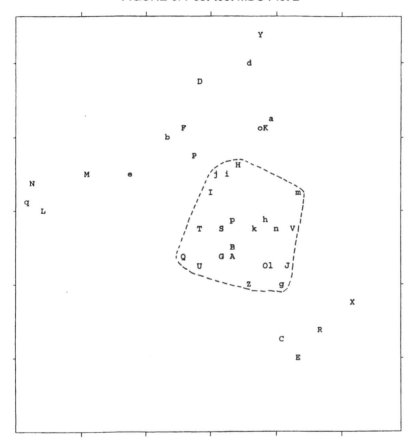

linkages, present in the intervention materials, have been formed in these posttest plots.

CONCLUSIONS

The cluster and MDS analysis of both the pretest and posttest data demonstrate that the risk clusters which were used to develop the pile sort stimuli are replicable domains, using this technique. This finding cross validates the results of our ethnographic interviewing. Additionally, this study demonstrates that the linkages between risks in one or more other risk areas can be successfully mapped using this technique, even when the stimuli are randomized and presented as individual risks.

The test results demonstrate that the boundaries between sub-groupings within a domain can be strengthened, and consequently some interconnections can be reduced or eliminated through time. New relationships can also be forged in the data, with concomitantly weaker boundaries and more interconnections. These conditions, creating a stronger boundary mechanism or establishing new linkages, support the utility of this method for the evaluation of prevention and intervention education programs focusing on drugs, alcohol, HIV, and other sexually transmitted diseases at a deep cognitive level.

It should be noted that these are preliminary findings. They are based on small numbers of students, and they were produced in situations where we had very little control over the external educational conditions that affect the students' awareness of the relationships between the risks. This pilot confirmation of the usefulness of the technique is stronger where the risks being explored did not interconnect in the pretest, but linked together in a posttest condition following an education program. The conclusion that we can promote from the data is that the pile sort process appears effective and produced enough defensible results to suggest that it be tried under far more controlled circumstances than those which prevailed in these tests. The process appears to have considerable promise for program evaluation efforts, and provides a possible mechanism for exploring the failure of an intervention program, as well as its success.

ENDNOTES

1. ANTHROPAC 4.0 (1993), by Steve Borgatti, is a program designed to assist in the collection and analysis of cognitive anthropology data sets such as free listings, pile sorts, and consensus theory. It also contains a number of programs for cluster analysis, unilinear scaling, multidimensional scaling, QAP, data management and transformations, and others. It is available from Analytic Technologies, 306 S. Walker St., Columbia, SC 29205.

2. NACA (Native Americans for Community Action) is a local non-profit organization that provides off-reservation services to Native Americans. These services include alcohol and drug counseling, health services, referral, and advocacy for social services. Other services include community educational programs, one of which is the AIDS prevention workshop featured in this pilot study.

REFERENCES CITED

Beauvais, F., Otting, E.R., Wolf, W. & Edwards, R.W (1989) American Indian Youth and Drugs, 1976-1987: A Continuing Problem. *American Journal of Public Health 79*(5), 634-636.

Blum, R.W., Harmon, B., Harris, L., Bergeisen, L. & Resnick M.D. (1992) American Indian–Alaska Native Youth Health. *Journal of the American Medical Association 267*(12), 1637-1644.

Boster, J.S. & Johnson, J.C. (1989) Form or Function: A Comparison of Expert and Novice Judgments of Similarity Among Fish. *American Anthropologist 91*(4), 866-889.

Kruskal, J.B. & Wish, M. (1978) Multi-Dimensional Scaling. Newbury Park, CA: Sage Publications.

Lamarine, R.J. (1988) Alcohol Abuse Among Native Americans. *Journal of Community Health 13*(3), 143-155.

Metler, R., Conway, G.A. & Stehr-Green, J. (1991) AIDS surveillance among American Indians and Alaska Natives. *American Journal of Public Health 81*(11), 1469-1479.

Roberts, J.M., Golder, T.V. & Chick, G.E. (1980) "Judgement, Oversight, and Skill: a cultural analysis of P-3 Pilot Error." *Human Organization 39*(1) 5-21.

Rolf, J., Alexander, C., Quintero, G., Trotter, R.T., Denetsosie, R., Tongue, N., Cha, D., Garcia, C. & Johnson, J. (1991a) *Findings from and innovative AIDS, alcohol, and other drug abuse prevention curriculum for Native American Youth*. Poster presented at the American Public Health Association's 119th Annual Meeting in Atlanta, Georgia.

Rolf, J., Baldwin, J., Trotter, R.T., Alexander, C., Denetsosie, R., Tongue, N., Quintero, G., Garcia, C. & Cha, D. (1991b) *Linking AIDS and AOD abuse prevention for Native American youth*. Poster presented at the Research Society on Alcoholism, Marco Island, Florida.

Toomey, K.E., Oberschelp, A.G. & Greenspan, J.R. (1989) Sexually Transmitted Diseases and Native Americans: Trends in Reported Gonorrhea and Syphilis Morbidity, 1984-1988. *Public Health Reports 104*(6), 566-572.

Trotter, R.T. II, Potter, J.M. & Price, L.J. (1993) AIDS and Ethnography: Advanced Ethnographic Research Methods for Exploring the HIV Epidemic. In D.A. Feldman ed. *AIDS and Anthropology in the United States*. Washington, D.C.: Am. Anth. Assoc.

Trotter, R.T. II, Rolf, J., Baldwin, J., Quintero, G.A. (In Press) Tough Issues for Navajo Youth and Navajo Schools. In J. Hanna, ed. *Tough Cases: School Outreach for At-Risk Youth*. Washington, D.C.: U.S. Department of Education.

Weller, S.C. & Romney, A.K. (1988) *Systematic Data Collection*. Newbury Park, CA: Sage Publications, Inc.

Contact Tracing for HIV Infection: Policy and Program Implications from a 50-State Survey

Geoffrey A. D. Smereck, AB, JD

SUMMARY. Contact tracing, the identification and active recruitment of non-self-presenting persons likely to be exposed to communicable disease, has been a major public health practice in the United States since the syphilis control programs of the 1940s. The nature of the AIDS epidemic, however, creates extraordinary difficulties for contact tracing programs attempting to reduce HIV infection. An analysis is here presented of the contact tracing strategies currently employed by the 50 States to combat the AIDS epidemic. Policy and programming implications are drawn from this 50-State survey, in an effort to adjust current contact tracing programs for HIV infection to improve their effectiveness.

INTRODUCTION

The Acquired Immunodeficiency Syndrome (AIDS) epidemic, the most dangerous public health crisis in American history, continues its horrific assault. The causative Human Immunodeficiency

Geoffrey A. D. Smereck is Vice President and Associate Project Director at Personalized Nursing Corporation, P.C., Plymouth, MI.

[Haworth co-indexing entry note]: "Contact Tracing for HIV Infection: Policy and Program Implications from a 50-State Survey." Smereck, Geoffrey A.D. Co-published simultaneously in *Drugs & Society* (The Haworth Press, Inc.) Vol. 7, No. 3/4, 1993, pp. 41-52; and: *AIDS and Community-Based Drug Intervention Programs: Evaluation and Outreach* (ed: Dennis G. Fisher, and Robert Needle) The Haworth Press, Inc., 1993, pp. 41-52. Multiple copies of this article/chapter may be purchased from The Haworth Document Delivery Center [1-800-3-HA-WORTH; 9:00 a.m. - 5:00 p.m. (EST)].

Copyright © 1993 by Taylor & Francis

Virus (HIV), which is transmitted via physical contact with infected blood and body fluids, continues to be spread primarily by the illicit drug-using activity of injecting drug users (IDUs) and by high-risk homosexual and heterosexual activity. Of the 213,641 diagnosed AIDS cases reported to the United States Centers for Disease Control (CDC), through February 1992, fully 90.4% derived from injecting drug use and high-risk sexual activity (CDC, March 1992, p. 8).

Yet vastly larger numbers of Americans are, today, HIV-infected and unaware of their predicament. Reliable data on the current number of asymptomatic HIV-positive Americans are unavailable; the most authoritative estimate places the number at 1.0 to 1.2 million as of late 1989 (CDC, 1990). Due to the extraordinarily long incubation period for AIDS, HIV-infected persons take an average of eight to eleven years to develop symptoms of diagnosable AIDS (Rutherford et al., 1990). In the absence of a vaccine or curative antiviral therapy, once symptoms of AIDS are present, the disease is thought by many to be 100% fatal, although 51% of the San Francisco male cohort who seroconverted (became HIV-positive) from 1977-1980 were still alive eleven years later (Rutherford et al., 1990).

Contact tracing, the identification, location, and active recruitment of non-self-presenting persons likely to be exposed to communicable disease, has been a major public health practice in the United States since the syphilis control programs of the 1940s (Rothenberg et al., 1984). Typically, once the source, asymptomatic patient is identified as a carrier of the disease, appropriate inquiry is made to identify the persons whose special relationships with the source patient place them in especially-acute risk of infection, such as sexual and needle-sharing partners. The at-risk partners are then personally contacted, notified of their risk of infection, and offered treatment or other intervention to reduce their risk of infection. Contact tracing, with mixed results, has been employed to combat epidemics of hepatitis B (Munday et al., 1983), chlamydia (Katz et al., 1988), and gonorrhea (Potterat et al., 1977). The nature of the AIDS epidemic, however, creates extraordinary difficulties for contact tracing programs attempting to reduce the spread of HIV infection.

SPECIAL DIFFICULTIES IN CONDUCTING CONTACT TRACING IN THE AIDS SETTING

The AIDS epidemic has distinctive features that vex contact tracing efforts.

Under-Diagnosed Nature of HIV Disease

Only a small fraction of HIV infection is currently being diagnosed in the United States (Rutherford et al., 1988). The most recent, official estimate of asymptomatic HIV-positive Americans is 1.0 to 1.2 million as of late 1989 (CDC, 1990). But even this estimate is speculative; no rigorous, direct study of the number of unknowing HIV-positive Americans is currently available.

Moreover, the significance of under-reporting looms even larger in high-prevalence urban areas. New York City, for example, has 37,952 diagnosed AIDS cases, by the most recent report (CDC, March 1992, p. 6); vastly more than this number are HIV-positive (Smith et al., 1991). Such enormous numbers of HIV-positive persons in close circulation, themselves unaware of their disease and their ability to infect others, create gargantuan logistical burdens for any contact tracing program. The capacity of HIV-positive persons, unknowingly, to infect others is colossal.

Extremely Long Incubation Period Before Onset of AIDS Symptoms

The best current understanding is that the average incubation period, between HIV infection and the onset of symptoms supporting an AIDS diagnosis, is eight to eleven years (Rutherford et al., 1990). Even this number is soft, however, because 19% of the San Francisco male cohort were not only still alive but also were still asymptomatic, 11.1 years after their seroconversion to HIV-positivity, with no clinical signs or symptoms of HIV infection (Rutherford et al., 1990, p. 1183). Thus, the outside time duration of the HIV/AIDS incubation period has not yet been clinically established. It follows that each HIV-positive person has an average of at least eight to eleven years (and more) to infect others.

High Mobility and Multiplicity of HIV Risk Partners

Most high-risk transmitters of HIV infection tend to have many, widely-dispersed, sex partners. In NIDA's recent study of drug use and sexual behaviors of the sex partners of IDUs, 24% of females and 40% of males had had sex with more than one partner in the prior six months (Weissman, 1991, p. 857). Likewise, CDC's very recent study of the AIDS sexual risk-taking activity of American high-school students has concluded that more than half of all high-school students in America "engage in behaviors that place them at risk for AIDS;" 29% of American high-school students have had four or more sex partners by senior year (CDC, April 1992). And in one of the few, documented studies of HIV contact tracing programs to date, only two generations of contact tracing identified 83 at-risk sex contacts from a single, HIV-positive source patient, and this in a rural, South Carolina community in only 24 months (Wykoff et al., 1988).

The logistical burden and expense of tracing and contacting even two generations of sex partners from all of the presently-known HIV-infected persons in high-prevalence areas, like New York City, would be astounding–and probably would absorb the bulk of the entire, current AIDS funding for such cities. Moreover, given the high mobility of HIV-infected IDUs and high-risk sexual partners, information discovered through contact tracing as to their location probably would not remain accurate for long; contact tracing information likely would remain current for only a small portion of any source patient's eight-to-eleven-year-plus period of infectivity.

Long Time Delay Between HIV Infection and the Ability to Detect the Infection

In the absence of any direct, clinical test for HIV, HIV infection can only be detected indirectly, by testing for the antibodies produced in reaction to HIV infection. The body produces these detectable antibodies only after a significant time delay after infection, which varies from six to twelve weeks or more (Ranki et al., 1987; Rutherford et al., 1990). The source patient remains contagious for the delay period. Thus even the best contact tracing programs will fail to trace the at-risk needle-sharing and sexual partners of HIV-infected persons who have not yet seroconverted.

Lack of Vaccine or Curative Antiviral Therapy

The present lack of an AIDS vaccine or curative antiviral therapy further blunts the effectiveness of contact tracing efforts. The voluntary citizen cooperation which is so necessary for effective contact tracing tends not to materialize, unless there is a widely-perceived benefit (such as a vaccine) that can justify so drastic an intrusion into the private lives of others. For example, contact tracing programs to combat the syphilis epidemic in the United States in the 1940s enjoyed the availability of a "magic bullet" remedy that would be dispensed to all at-risk persons traced by the program: penicillin. In contrast, the AIDS epidemic's absence of a "magic bullet" remedy has meant that little citizen participation will assist contact tracing efforts.

Importance of Maintaining Confidentiality

To an extent unprecedented in the history of epidemics, the AIDS epidemic coincided with a strong and pervasive societal demand for confidentiality. Confidentiality of HIV-positive identities has been justified on the ground of protecting source patients and their contacts from cruel discrimination and ostracism, leading to loss of employment, loss of insurance, even vigilantism. Moreover, as a practical matter, confidentiality of HIV-positive patient information has been thought essential to achieve the voluntary cooperation required for public health interventions (Becker, 1988; Becker et al., 1988; Brandt, 1988).

Reinforcing this, the lower federal courts have held that a Constitutional right of privacy protects people known or suspected of having HIV disease.[1] The decision of the United States Supreme Court in *Whalen v. Roe*,[2] though not directly involving HIV or AIDS, has been interpreted broadly to support a general Constitutional right to privacy of medical records, which requires both a limitation of access to public health officials who have a need to know, and also adequate protection of the confidentiality of record contents. An increasing number of court cases are upholding damage awards to compensate for violation of confidentiality concerning HIV-positivity.[3] Similarly, the States which have enacted contact tracing legislation for HIV infection also have enacted laws specifically protecting the confidentiality of the HIV-positive case record and related information.

SPECIAL NEEDS FOR CONTACT TRACING IN THE AIDS SETTING

Given the many, intrinsic difficulties of conducting contact tracing programs in the AIDS epidemic, it is inviting to reject such programs altogether. Yet the AIDS epidemic also presents a special need for contact tracing, in light of recent findings.

Sexual Partners and IDUs Generally Cannot Be Relied Upon to Notify Their At-Risk Partners of Their HIV Infection

In a recent, multi-site study of HIV-positive IDUs and their sexual partners, 19% either incorrectly reported their test results or incorrectly stated that they had not been tested at all (McCusker et al., 1992). In another recent study, low-income Hispanic men who were HIV-positive and who knew of their seropositivity were studied to determine if they had told their sexual partners of their HIV status. An alarming 52% had kept their HIV infection secret from one or more sexual partners (Marks et al., 1991).

These alarming findings contradict earlier, general studies of IDU self-report reliability, which had found fair agreement between self-reports and information shown in official records. However, these general studies were not in the AIDS context (Bonito et al., 1976).

Notification of HIV-Positivity Helps Change AIDS-Risk Behaviors

The weight of the research to date is that notification of a person's HIV infection assists significantly in bringing about change in the person's high-risk AIDS behaviors. In a recent study of New

York City blood donors who were notified they were HIV-positive, 60% significantly decreased their high-risk sexual behaviors after notification (Cleary et al., 1991). Similarly, other researchers have found that notification of HIV-positivity is associated with significant decreases in high-risk behaviors, compared to persons who have tested HIV-negative or who have not been tested (Fox et al., 1987). The research on this point, however, is not unanimous (Calsyn et al., 1992).

Notification of HIV-Infection Is Likely to Delay the Onset of AIDS Symptoms

Recent epidemiological research has shown that morphine, cocaine, and heroin speed the growth of HIV in cultures of human immune cells (Peterson et al., 1990; Peterson et al., 1991). If, as this research indicates, morphine, cocaine, and heroin are actual co-factors in the growth of HIV within the human immune system, the continued use of such drugs by IDUs after their HIV-positivity seriously exacerbates their HIV disease, and may well increase AIDS mortality and shorten the incubation period before AIDS symptoms.

STATE CONTACT TRACING PROGRAMS FOR HIV INFECTION AND PARTNER NOTIFICATION

The 39 States which by legislation have adopted some form of HIV contact tracing have addressed these special difficulties and special needs, in various ways.

Mandatory/Voluntary Disclosure of Known Contacts

Most contact tracing States have finessed the issue whether or not to mandate reporting and name notification of partner HIV-positive persons. They generally mandate contact tracing efforts by county or state public health officers (PHO) employed by official health departments, as long as the identities of at-risk partners already have been provided to the health department. Also, they usually mandate the reporting to the PHO, by physicians or testing laboratories, of non-identifying, epidemiological information on all persons who receive an HIV-positive test result. The majority of States, however, do not go further to mandate that physicians or other health care professionals notify third parties who are at risk of being HIV-infected by the source patient, even if the identities of at-risk partners are fully known and they are easily contacted. Ten states (AZ, CA, CT, IA, IL, MI, PA, NY, VA, WV) have gone so far as to declare there is no duty on the part of the physicians or health care providers to warn known at-risk partners.

Confidentiality Issues

The contact tracing States generally have made great efforts to protect the confidentiality of HIV-positive source patient information. Five states (CT, LA, MI, NY, PA) require that the physician or PHO make the notification to at-risk partners "in person," or "face-to-face," unless circumstances reasonably prevent doing so. Fourteen states (AZ, CA, CT, FL, IL, IN, KY, LA, MD, MI, MT, NY, RI, WI) require the physician or PHO, prior to disclosure, to attempt through counseling to have the source patient notify his/her sexual and drug partners.

Fifteen states (AL, CA, CO, FL, GA, ID, IN, KS, MI, NH, NY, ND, RI, UT, WI) make unauthorized disclosure of HIV-positivity a crime (13 states, a misdemeanor; two states, ND and NH, a felony; the most serious category of crimes punishable by more than one year in prison). Thirteen states (AZ, DE, HI, IA, KY, LA, ME, MO, NJ, OR, VT, VA, WV) make unauthorized disclosure of HIV status a lesser, civil infraction, although punishable by monetary fines of up to $10,000 (HI, NJ).

Four states (CT, GA, LA, NY) require that the physician or PHO must specifically notify the HIV-positive source patient of his/her intent to notify the source patient's partner, prior to the notification. Two states (NY, LA) require that the source patient be given the option of having the disclosure of his/her HIV-positivity be made by a physician or a PHO, at the patient's choice. Ten states (CT, LA, NY, KS, SC, MT, NH, IN, WV, NJ) expressly mandate that specific identifying information of the source patient not be disclosed to the notified partners; partners are told only that there is reason to believe that a past or present sex or drug partner is HIV-positive. Twelve states (AZ, CA, FL, GA, IL, KS, KY, MO, OH, RI, TX, WV) specially authorize notification of spouses.

Abrogation of Health Professionals' Common Law Duty to Warn Third-Parties in Danger

A striking feature of many of the State contact tracing programs for HIV infection is their nullification of the common law duty, traditionally placed upon physicians, psychiatrists, and similar health professionals, to warn known third-parties of a foreseeable danger to them from a patient. The classic illustration is provided by *Tarasoff v. Regents of University of California*,[4] in which the California Supreme Court held that psychotherapists have an affirmative duty to warn a third-party of the foreseeable danger from their patients. The patient, during the course of therapy, had confided his intention to kill a third-party, but the psychotherapists did not contact the third-party to warn her, even though her identity and location had been disclosed by the patient. The patient in fact murdered her. The *Tarasoff* court ruled that, given the foreseeability of the danger, the severity of the harm to the third-party, and the ease by which the warning could have been made, the psychotherapists had had a common law duty to contact the third-party to warn her of the danger.[5]

In this spirit, a long line of cases has held physicians to be under a duty to warn third parties of specific risks to them from patients with smallpox, tuberculosis, syphilis, typhus, meningitis, scarlet fever, and diphtheria.[6]

In stark contrast to this traditional common law duty, many of the contact tracing States have undercut their programs by granting extraordinary immunity from liability if health care professionals fail to contact known at-risk partners of HIV-infected patients. It is difficult to justify this grant of immunity on public health grounds. Ironically, it even contradicts the policy of the American Medical Association, which requires physicians as a matter of professional ethics to notify sexual and drug-sharing partners of their risk of HIV infection, if their infected patients refuse to do so (AMA, 1988).

Rather, physicians and similar health care professionals are the best-positioned to intervene effectively via contact tracing. Over half (52%) of all adults in the United States who were HIV-tested in 1988 received their testing through a physician (Hardy et al., 1990). Moreover, they are the professionals who are most likely to learn the identities of at-risk partners of HIV-infected persons. It is a mistake to nullify their common law duty to warn.

CONCLUSIONS

The special nature of the AIDS epidemic presents extraordinary difficulties for contact tracing programs in the United States attempting to reduce the spread of HIV infection. The 39 States which, by legislation, have created contact tracing programs, have deferred to the political exigencies as much as the epidemiological ones. They, to a significant extent, have de-emphasized compulsory notification of sexual and drug-sharing partners of HIV-positive persons, have emphasized anonymity of reporting, strongly have protected the confidentiality of HIV-positive patients and their sexual and drug-sharing partners, and have abrogated the common law duty to warn known, at-risk third-parties which the States have imposed upon physicians and other health care professionals for many generations. This general nullification of health care professionals' duty to warn known, easily-notified third-parties of foreseeable, life-threatening danger, seems unwarranted in the AIDS context, cannot be justified on public health or patient-protection grounds, and undercuts the efficacy of the contact tracing programs of the States.

ENDNOTES

1. *Doe v. Borough of Barrington*, 729 F. Supp 376 (D.N.J. 1990); *Woods v. White*, 689 F. Supp 874 (W. D. Wis. 1988); *Doe v. Coughlin*, 697 F. Supp 1234 (N.D.N.Y 1988).

2. *Whalen v. Roe*, 429 US 589, 602 and n.29 (1977).

3. *Estate of Urbaniak v. Newton*, 277 Cal. Rptr. 354, 226 C.A.3d 1128 (1991); *Beason v. Harclerod*, 105 Ore. App. 376 (1991); *Estate of Behringer v. Princeton Medical Center*, 249 N. J. Super. 597, 592 A.2d 1251 (1991); *Hilman v. Columbia County*, 164 Wis.2d 376, 474 N.W. 2d 913 (1991).

4. *Tarasoff v. Regents of University of California*, 131 Cal. Rptr. 14, 551 P.2d 334 (Calif. 1976).

5. 551 P.2d at 347-348 (Calif. 1976).
6. *Shepard v. Redford Community Hospital*, 390 N.W.2d 239 (Mich.Ct.App. 1986); *Fosgate v. Corona*, 330 A.2d 355 (N.J. 1974); *Hoffman v. Blackmon*, 241 So.2d 752 (Fla. Ct. App. 1970); *Jones v. Stanko*, 160 N.E. 456 (Ohio 1928); *Davis v. Rodman*, 227 S.W. 612 (Ark. 1921); *Skillings v. Allen*, 173 N.W. 663 (Minn. 1919); *State v. Wordin*, 14 A. 801 (Conn. 1887).

REFERENCES

American Medical Association (1988). *HIV blood test counseling: AMA physician guidelines.*
Becker, M. H. (1988). AIDS and behavior change. *Public Health Review, 16,* 1-11.
Becker, M. H., & Joseph, J. G. (1988). AIDS and behavior change to reduce risk: a review. *American Journal of Public Health, 78,* 394-410.
Bonito, A. J., Nurco, D. N., Shaffer, J. W. (1976). The veridicality of addicts' self-reports in social research. *International Journal of Addictions, 11,* 719-724.
Brandt, A. M. (1988). AIDS in historical perspective: Four lessons from the history of sexually transmitted diseases. *American Journal of Public Health, 78,* 367-371.
Calsyn, D. A., Saxon, A. J., Freeman, G., Whittaker, S. (1992). Ineffectiveness of AIDS education and HIV antibody testing in reducing high-risk behaviors among injecting drug users. *American Journal of Public Health, 82,* 573-575.
Centers for Disease Control (1990). Estimates of HIV prevalence and projected AIDS cases: Summary of a workshop, October 31-November 1, 1989. *Morbidity and Mortality Weekly Report, 39,* 110-2, 117-9.
Centers for Disease Control (1992, March). *HIV/AIDS Surveillance Report,* Atlanta, GA U.S. Department of Health & Human Services.
Centers for Disease Control (1992, April). Teen-agers and AIDS: the risk worsens. *New York Times,* April 14, 1992, p. B6.
Cleary, P. D., Devanter, N. V., Rogers, T. F., Singer, E., Shipton-Levy, R., Steilen, M., Stuart, A., Avorn, J., Pindyck, J. (1991). Behavior changes after notification of HIV infection. *American Journal of Public Health, 81,* 1586-1590.
Fox, R., Odaka, N. J., Brookmeyer, R., Polk, B. F. (1987). Effect of HIV antibody disclosure on subsequent sexual activity in homosexual men. *AIDS, 1,* 241-246.
Hardy, A. M., & Dawson, D. A. (1990). HIV antibody testing among adults in the United States: Data from 1988 NHIS. *American Journal of Public Health, 80,* 586-589.
Katz, B. P., Danos, C. S., Quinn, T. S. (1988). Efficiency and cost-effectiveness of field follow-up for patients with *Chlamydia Trachomatis* infection in a sexually transmitted disease clinic. *Sexually Transmitted Diseases, 15,* 11-16.
Marks, G., Richardson, J. L., Maldonado, N. (1991). Self-disclosure of HIV

infection to sexual partners. *American Journal of Public Health, 81,* 1321-1323.

McCusker, J., Stoddard, A. M., McCarthy, E. (1992). The validity of self-reported HIV antibody test results. *American Journal of Public Health, 82,* 567-569.

Munday, P. E., McDonald, W., Murray-Sykes, K. M. (1983). Contact tracing in hepatitis B. *British Journal of Venereal Disease, 59,* 314-316.

Peterson, P., Sharp, B., Gekker, G. (1990). Morphine promotes the growth of HIV-1 in human peripheral blood mononuclear cell co-cultures. *AIDS, 4,* 869-873.

Peterson, P., Gekker, G., Chao, C., Schut, R. (1991). Cocaine potentiates HIV-1 replication in human peripheral blood mononuclear cell cocultures. *Journal of Immunology, 146,* 81-84.

Potterat, J. J., & Rothenberg, R. B. (1977). The case-finding effectiveness of a self-referral system for gonorrhea: A preliminary report. *American Journal of Public Health, 67,* 174-176.

Ranki, A., Valle, S. L., Krohn, M. (1987, Sept. 12). Long latency precedes overt seroconversion in sexually transmitted human immunodeficiency virus infection. *Lancet,* 589-593.

Rothenberg, R. B., & Potterat, J. J. (1984). Strategies for management of sex partners. In Holmes, K.K., Mardh, P.A. et al. (Eds.), *Sexually Transmitted Diseases,* pp. 965-972. New York: McGraw-Hill International Book Co.

Rutherford, G. W., & Woo, J. M. (1988). Editorial: Contact tracing and the control of human immunodeficiency virus infection. *Journal of the American Medical Association, 259,* 3609-10.

Rutherford, G. W., Lifson, A. R., Hessol, N. A., Darrow, W. W., O'Mally, P. M., Buchbinder, S. P., Barnhart, J. L., Bodecker, T. W., Cannon, L., Doll, L. S., Holmberg, S. D., Harrison, J. S., Roger, M. F., Werdegar, D., Jaffe, H. W. (1990, November). Course of HIV-1 infection in a cohort of homosexual and bisexual men: An 11-year follow-up study. *British Medical Journal, 301,* 1183-1188.

Smith, P. F., Mikl, J., Hyde, S., Morse, D. L. (1991, May). The AIDS epidemic in New York State. *American Journal of Public Health, 81 Supp,* 54-60.

Weissman, G. (1991, December 13). Drug use and sexual behaviors among sex partners of injecting drug users–United States, 1988-1990. *Morbidity and Mortality Weekly Report, 40,* 857.

Wykoff, R. F., Health, C. W., Hollis, S. L. (1988). Contact tracing to identify human immunodeficiency virus infection in a rural community. *Journal of the American Medical Association, 259,* 3563-3566.

A Comparison
of HIV Related Risk Behaviors
# of Street Recruited
and Treatment Program
Recruited Injection Drug Users

Dale D. Chitwood, PhD
James R. Rivers, PhD
Mary Comerford, MSPH
Duane C. McBride, PhD

SUMMARY. This paper compares the demographic traits and the risk behaviors of injection drug users (IDUs) not in treatment who were recruited into an AIDS risk reduction program in Miami, FL with attributes of IDUs who were clients of drug treatment programs. The majority of both IDU samples were male and in their 30's. Most street IDUs were African-American; a majority of treatment clients were White, non-Hispanic. Prevalence of HIV was high

Dale D. Chitwood, James R. Rivers, and Mary Comerford are affiliated with the School of Medicine at University of Miami. Duane C. McBride is affiliated with Andrews University.

This research was supported by NIDA Grants DA04433 and DA06910.

Requests for reprints should be sent to Dale D. Chitwood, University of Miami, 1400 N.W. 10th Avenue, Room 210 A, Miami, FL 33136.

[Haworth co-indexing entry note]: "A Comparison of HIV Related Risk Behaviors of Street Recruited and Treatment Program Recruited Injection Drug Users." Chitwood, Dale D. et al. Co-published simultaneously in *Drugs & Society* (The Haworth Press, Inc.) Vol. 7, No. 3/4, 1993, pp. 53-63; and: *AIDS and Community-Based Drug Intervention Programs: Evaluation and Outreach* (ed: Dennis G. Fisher, and Richard Needle), The Haworth Press, Inc., 1993, pp. 53-63. Multiple copies of this article/chapter may be purchased from The Haworth Document Delivery Center [1-800-3-HAWORTH; 9:00 a.m. - 5:00 p.m. (EST)].

Copyright © 1993 by Taylor & Francis

for African-Americans and Hispanics from both IDU samples. Prevalence of HIV was relatively low among both samples of White, non-Hispanic IDUs but somewhat higher among White street IDUs than among White treatment clients. Similar proportions of street and treatment IDUs injected daily, but street IDUs were more likely to share works, inject in shooting galleries, use crack and alcohol daily, have multiple sex partners and have IDU sex partners.

Strategies to prevent the spread of HIV were initiated at the federal level during the 1980's, and in 1987 the National Institute on Drug Abuse (NIDA) established targeted outreach demonstration projects designed to intervene with high risk injection drug users (IDUs) (McBride, Chitwood, Page, McCoy, & Inciardi, 1990). These National AIDS Demonstration Research (NADR) projects had four related tasks. The first was to identify a population of IDUs who were at high risk for exposure/transmission of HIV. The three associated tasks were to develop risk reduction intervention programs, to implement those programs among the high risk IDU population, and to evaluate the efficacy of those programs.

The demonstration projects implemented their intervention programs among street IDUs who were not clients of drug treatment programs. This population was chosen because street IDUs were considered to be at a very high risk for HIV and to be without access to risk reduction programs.

The decision to target the street IDU subpopulation was not a simple task. At the time of the selection of the target population, various subpopulations were known to exist within the larger population of IDUs, but most of the published research about IDUs was dominated by studies of institutionally associated populations such as drug treatment clients, incarcerated IDUs, and to a lesser extent, emergency room patients (Cavanaugh, Ginzburg, Harwood, Hubbard, Marsden, & Rachal, 1989; Chitwood & Chitwood, 1981; Inciardi, McBride, Pottieger, Russe, & Siegel, 1978; O'Donnell, 1969). Although it was believed that street IDUs exhibited more high risk behavior, the urgency of the AIDS crisis required the implementation of the NADR projects before studies could be completed which compared the risk behaviors of drug treatment clients with those of IDUs who were not in treatment.

The purpose of this paper is to investigate whether IDUs who had no recent treatment experience and who had been recruited from the streets of Dade County, Florida into a NADR demonstration project (street IDUs) were more likely to engage in high risk HIV related behaviors than were IDUs who were clients of drug treatment programs that were located within the same catchment areas (treatment IDUs). This comparison will help answer the question: "Should intervention programs continue to target IDUs who are not in drug treatment?"

METHOD

Subjects

The data reported in this paper were obtained from 464 IDUs who were clients of drug treatment programs and 1022 street recruited IDUs who were not in treatment. These two distinct samples of IDUs were enrolled in separate research projects in Dade County, Florida. The treatment sample was drawn from a panel study of IDUs who were in drug treatment at the time of study enrollment, and the street sample was from the Miami NADR project whose participants were not in treatment. The panel study of the epidemiology of HIV among IDUs in drug treatment was initiated in April, 1987, and in October of that year the Miami NADR project was funded (Chitwood, Comerford, Anderson, Ross, & Fishwick, 1990; Chitwood, Inciardi et al., 1991; McCoy & Khoury, 1990). All study participants in both research projects gave informed consent, were interviewed, received a small stipend for their participation, received HIV pretest counseling, had blood drawn by venipuncture for laboratory analyses, and were provided HIV test results and posttest counseling.

Treatment Recruited Subjects

Between May, 1987 and August, 1988, 604 individuals who were enrolled in drug treatment in Miami, Florida and had injected one or more drugs some time since January, 1978 were recruited at their treatment program into a panel study designed to assess the incidence and prevalence of HIV. A structured interview was administered to all participants at their treatment center in a private one-to-one setting by trained interviewers who were not part of the treatment facility staff. All participants were assured that their data would not be disclosed to anyone including the staff of the treatment programs. Questions about demographic traits and drug use history, injection behaviors, and sexual history during the past year were included in the interview.

Of the 604 Miami treatment clients enrolled in that study, 464 had injected drugs within twelve months prior to their interview. In order to approximate an injection time frame that more closely coincided with the use period of the street recruited IDU study participants of the NADR project, only the data collected from those 464 IDUs are included in this article.

Street Recruited Subjects

Between March, 1988 and February, 1990, 1022 IDUs were recruited from the streets by outreach workers into the Miami NADR project, which employed a snowball sampling design to access several networks of IDUs. Eligibility requirements included drug injection during the six months prior to enrollment and no history of drug treatment during that six month period. After being screened on the street by outreach staff, subjects were re-screened at an assessment center where eligible IDUs were interviewed with the AIDS Initial Assessment (AIA) instrument. Demographic, drug use, injection, and sex behavior histories for the six months prior to interview were collected by trained interviewers in confidential one-to-one sessions.

Interview Instruments

Each study used a separate instrument, but many questions were the same or yielded comparable information. The major difference in the two instruments was the "time at risk" which was assessed by the behavior questions. The treatment-recruited sample was asked about activities that occurred in the previous twelve months while the street-recruited sample reported behavior that occurred in the past six months. Compared to data reported by the treatment client IDU sample, this difference in risk period probably produced from the street-recruited IDUs a conservative estimate of certain risk behaviors, such as the number of sex partners reported by the street-recruited NADR sample.

Because the primary question of this paper is whether street-recruited IDUs who are not in treatment are at greater risk for HIV exposure/transmission than are IDUs recruited from drug treatment programs, the observed differences in risk behavior that are produced by these interview instruments provide a conservative answer. If street-recruited IDUs report more risk behavior in six months than treatment client IDUs report in twelve months, it is reasonable to assume that these reported differences are real.

RESULTS

Demographics

The demographic traits of the street and the treatment IDU samples are reported in Table 1. Three quarters (74.9%) of the street and nearly two thirds (64.7%) of the treatment IDUs were male. Approximately half (48.4%) of the street IDUs and nearly as many (42.5%) treatment clients were at least 35 years old. Street IDUs (60.8%) were less likely than treatment clients (78.7%) to have a high school diploma or GED. No differences in employment status were observed; approximately half of both groups were unemployed. Nine out of ten (88.7%) street IDUs and three out of four (74.4%) treatment IDUs had a history of incarceration.

The major demographic difference between the two IDU groups was ethnicity. The street sample was predominantly African-American (70.7%), while the majority of the treatment sample were White, non-Hispanic (62.5%). Slightly more than one out of every ten members of each IDU group were Hispanic.

HIV Status

One third (32.6%) of the street IDUs and 17.0 percent of the treatment group tested positive for antibodies to HIV (Table 1). When ethnic specific levels of HIV prevalence were calculated,

Table 1

Socio-Demographic Characteristics of Street and Treatment
Injection Drug Users

Characteristic	IDU Group		
	Street N = 1022	Treatment N = 464	X^2
	(%)	(%)	
Male	74.9	64.7	16.35****
35 or Older	48.4	42.5	4.58*
High School Diploma/GED	60.8	78.7	45.80****
Currently Unemployed	51.1	46.3	2.87
Ever Incarcerated	88.7	74.4	51.61****
Ethnicity			
African-American	70.7	21.3	315.16****
Hispanic	11.0	14.7	4.10
White, non-Hispanic	17.6	62.5	297.34****
Other Ethnic Groups	0.7	1.5	a
HIV Ab +			
All	32.6	17.0	38.54****
African-American	37.2	37.4	0.0
Hispanic	30.6	27.9	0.12
White, non-Hispanic	15.0	7.9	5.84*

*p < .05. **p < .01. ***p < .001. ****p < .0001.
a Number too few to calculate X^2.

however, this difference largely disappeared. Both the street IDUs
(37.2%) and treatment clients (37.4%) of African American heri-
tage had similarly high HIV prevalence levels, as did street (30.6%)
and treatment (27.9%) IDUs of Hispanic origin. Only the White,
non-Hispanic street users (15.0%) had a significantly higher preva-

lence of HIV than did their treatment client counterparts (7.9%), although prevalence among both of these groups was comparatively low.

Drug Use Behaviors

One half (54.3%) of the street IDUs and two thirds (67.9%) of the treatment clients began to inject drugs prior to 1976. Relatively few IDUs from either sample recently had initiated injection, although a higher percentage of street (23.0%) than treatment IDUs (14.3%) first injected after 1981 (Table 2). This observation was true for African-American and White, non-Hispanic IDUs, but among IDUs of Hispanic origin, street IDUs were no more likely than treatment clients to have initiated use after 1981 (data not shown).

Similar proportions of street (45.1%) and treatment (43.5%) IDUs injected drugs at least once per day, but street IDUs were more likely to use non-injectable drugs (Table 2). Whereas three

Table 2

Drug Use and Injection Behaviors of Street and Treatment Injection Drug Users

Behavior	IDU Group		
	Street $\underline{N}$ = 1022	Treatment $\underline{N}$ = 464	X^2
	(%)	(%)	
Initiated injection BEFORE 1976	54.3	67.9	24.26****
Initiated injection AFTER 1981	23.0	14.3	11.26***
Injecting daily	45.1	43.5	0.57
Smoking crack	76.9	42.0	173.07****
Smoking crack daily	35.0	14.4	66.25****
Drinking alcohol daily	32.6	17.0	38.54****

*$\underline{p}$ < .05. **$\underline{p}$ < .01. ***$\underline{p}$ < .001. ****$\underline{p}$ < .0001.

quarters (76.9%) of the street IDUs had smoked crack during the past six months and 35.0 percent smoked crack daily, only 42.0 percent of the treatment IDUs had smoked crack during the past year and 14.4 percent smoked crack daily. Street IDUs (32.6%) similarly were nearly twice as likely as treatment IDUs (17.0%) to drink alcohol daily. These associations also were observed within each ethnic specific group (data not shown).

HIV Related Risk Behavior

The HIV related high risk behaviors of street IDUs are compared with those of treatment client IDUs in Table 3, and high risk injection and sex behaviors were reported more often by street IDUs. Needle sharing was extensive within each IDU sample. Three quarters (75.2%) of the street IDUs and two thirds (65.7%) of the treatment IDUs reported that they shared injection equipment. Injection in shooting galleries was reported more than twice as often by street

Table 3

High Risk Injection and Sex Behavior of Street and Treatment Injection Drug Users

Behavior	IDU GROUP		
	Street $\underline{N}$ = 1022	Treatment $\underline{N}$ = 464	X^2
	(%)	(%)	
Sharing needles	75.2	65.7	14.41****
Injecting in Shooting Galleries	42.7	18.3	83.05****
Multiple Sex Partners	72.8	48.5	83.11****
IDU Sex Partners	58.6	50.0	9.6 **
Condom Use	42.0	29.7	19.52****

*$\underline{p}$ < .05. **$\underline{p}$ < .01. ***$\underline{p}$ < .001. ****$\underline{p}$ < .0001.

IDUs who were not in treatment (42.7%) than by treatment IDUs (18.3%).

African American, Hispanic, and White, Non-Hispanic street IDUs were more likely than their treatment counterparts to report needle sharing and injection in a shooting gallery (data not shown).

Street IDUs who were recruited into the NADR project were considerably more likely (72.8%) than drug treatment IDUs (48.5%) to report they had multiple sex partners. Street IDUs (58.6%) also were somewhat more likely than treatment clients (50.0%) to report that at least one of their sex partners was an IDU. Condoms infrequently were used by either sample of IDUs, but street IDUs (42.0%) were more likely than treatment IDUs (29.7%) to have used a condom on at least one occasion. These relationships were unchanged for African Americans, Hispanics and White, non-Hispanics (data not shown).

DISCUSSION

The major finding of this investigation is that IDUs who were not in drug treatment and who were recruited from the streets into a NADR intervention project were more likely than IDUs who were clients of drug treatment programs located within the same urban setting, to report high risk injection and high risk sex behaviors, in spite of the fact that the risk exposure period for the street IDUs was half that of the risk period for treatment client IDUs. Street IDUs definitely are at high risk for HIV exposure/transmission. These findings strongly support the decision of the NADR projects to target their HIV related risk behavior reduction programs among street IDUs who were not enrolled in a formal drug treatment program.

Not only did the NADR study access very high risk street IDUs who were members of the three largest ethnic communities of Miami, but the majority of its enrollees also were members of ethnic groups who had HIV infection levels that were two to three times that of the White, non-Hispanic IDUs who constituted the majority of the drug treatment sample. Projects like NADR that recruit from the street are likely to enroll many IDUs who are in need of early intervention for HIV related disease and who are at high risk for HIV transmission to their sex partners and to other IDUs.

This study compared IDUs from two specific recruitment sources: (a) volunteer study participants who were not in drug treatment and who were recruited from the street, and (b) volunteer respondents who were recruited at drug treatment programs into a study that was not associated with any treatment or HIV risk reduction program. The observed differences may be influenced to some extent by the recruitment source. A recent study which recruited IDUs only from the street and dichotomized street-recruited participants into drug treatment client IDU and not in drug treatment IDU groups, did not find major differences between treatment clients and other IDUs (Alcabes, Vlahov, & Anthony, 1992). If street-recruitable treatment clients engage in risk behaviors that are more like the behaviors of IDUs who are not in treatment than they are like the behaviors of other treatment clients who cannot be recruited from the street environment, then street recruitment into HIV risk behavior reduction programs should be expanded to include treatment clients who are active IDUs as well as IDUs who are participating in a formal treatment program.

The decision to target out-of-treatment IDUs does not preclude the importance of providing risk reduction intervention in treatment programs. Although treatment clients were less likely than street IDUs to report high risk injection and sex behaviors, many clients engaged in risky activities and were in need of intervention services.

Nevertheless, specific characteristics of the street IDU and the treatment client IDU samples reported in this study support the conclusion that out-of-treatment IDUs are more likely to engage in high risk activities. It is interesting to note that street and treatment client IDUs were equally likely to inject drugs daily but street IDUs were more likely to share injection equipment and to inject at shooting galleries. It appears that frequency of injection does not account for high risk sharing practices.

Furthermore, the fact that street IDUs also were more likely to have multiple sex partners and to have IDU sex partners suggests that street IDUs generally may live more risk-filled lives. There is reason to expect that treatment IDUs would be influenced by the treatment setting to engage in less risky injection behaviors than do IDUs who are not in treatment, but there is less reason to expect that treatment IDUs who had never been counseled or tested for HIV would be influenced by the treatment program to engage in less risky sexual activities. Regardless of the reasons, the data support the decision to target out-of-treatment street IDUs with AIDS risk reduction demonstration projects.

REFERENCES

Alcabes, P., Vlahov, D. & Anthony, J.C. (1992). Correlates of human immunodeficiency virus infection in intravenous drug users: are treatment-program samples misleading? *British Journal of Addiction, 87,* 47-54.

Chitwood, D.D. & Chitwood, J.S. (1981). A Comparison of officially defined drug abusers and individuals with self-identified drug use problems. *The International Journal of Addictions, 16*(5), 909-923.

Chitwood, D.D., Comerford, M., Anderson, R., Ross, S.D., Fishwick, J. (1990). Prevalence and incidence of human immunodeficiency virus type 1 (HIV-1) among intravenous drug users in South Florida. *American Journal of Epidemiology, 132*(4), 771.

Chitwood, D.D., Inciardi, J.A., McBride, D.C., McCoy, C.B., McCoy, H.V. & Trapido, E.J. (1991). *A community approach to AIDS intervention.* New York: Greenwood Press.

Hubbard, R.L., Marsden, M.E. & Rachal, J., Harwood, H.J., Cavanaugh, E.R. & Ginzburg, H.M. (1989). *Drug abuse treatment.* Chapel Hill: The University of North Carolina Press.

Inciardi, J.A., McBride, D.C., Pottieger, A.E., Russe, B.R. & Siegel, H.A. (1978). *Legal and illicit drugs: Acute reactions of emergency room populations.* New York: Holt, Rinehart & Winston.

McBride, D.C., Chitwood, D.D., Page, J.B., McCoy, C.B. & Inciardi, J.A. (1990). AIDS, IV drug use, and the federal agenda. In J.A. Inciardi (Ed.), *Handbook of drug control in the United States* (pp. 267-282). New York: Greenwood Press.

McCoy, C.B. & Khoury, E. (1990). Drug use and the risk of AIDS. *American Behavioral Scientist, 33,* 419-431.

O'Donnell, J.A. (1969). *Narcotic addicts in Kentucky.* PHS Publication (No. 1881). Washington, DC: U.S. Government Printing Office.

Social Network Structures:
An Ethnographic Analysis
of Intravenous Drug Use
in Houston, Texas

Mark L. Williams, PhD
Jay Johnson, MA, MS

One of the major frustrations of research on the transmission of Human Immunodeficiency Virus (HIV) infection among intravenous drug abusers has been an inability to fully explain the wide variety of behaviors and social conditions which have been found to be associated with increased risk of HIV infection among drug injectors in differing locations throughout the United States (Alperin, & Needle, 1991; Woodhouse, Patterat, Klovdahl, Darrow, Muth, & Muth, J., 1990). A recent summary of characteristics and behaviors of intravenous drug users found to be associated with HIV seropositivity in low seroprevalence areas reported no less than seven factors (Siegal, Carlson, Falck et al., 1991). In addition, the authors found two social and behavioral characteristics associated with serostatus in their sample that were previously unreported. In

Mark L. Williams and Jay Johnson are associated with Affiliated Systems Corporation in Houston, TX.

[Haworth co-indexing entry note]: "Social Network Structures: An Ethnographic Analysis of Intravenous Drug Use in Houston, Texas." Williams, Mark L., and Jay Johnson. Co-published simultaneously in *Drugs & Society* (The Haworth Press, Inc.) Vol. 7, No. 3/4, 1993, pp. 65-90; and: *AIDS and Community-Based Drug Intervention Programs: Evaluation and Outreach* (ed: Dennis G. Fisher, & Richard Needle), The Haworth Press, Inc., 1993, pp. 65-90. Multiple copies of this article/chapter may be purchased from The Haworth Document Delivery Center [1-800-3-HAWORTH; 9:00 a.m. - 5:00 p.m. (EST)].

Copyright © 1993 by Taylor & Francis

an attempt to form a more parsimonious explanation, geographic variation in seroprevalence rates among drug injectors have been related to at least three factors: time of introduction of the virus into an intravenous drug using population; racial characteristics of a population; and duration and activities of HIV infection prevention efforts (Friedman, Quimby, Sufian, Abdul-Quader, & Des Jarlais, 1989; Watters, 1988). Yet, there is at least a tacit recognition that these factors fail to adequately explain observed variation. For example, the time of introduction of a virus into a population would make little difference in observed seroprevalence rates over time; there is no evidence to suggest that any particular racial group is more susceptible to HIV infection than another; and HIV prevention efforts seem to produce few observable variations in outcomes between samples of drug users participating in minimal and extensive prevention efforts.

Watters (1988; 1989) offers a far more satisfying explanation of the variation in seroprevalence rates among populations of intravenous drug users. This explanation proposes that the context of intravenous drug use will account for seroprevalence variation. Context is defined as the conditions in which a population of drug users inject. Context as an explanation of varying rates of HIV infection does have an intuitive appeal. For example, the rates of HIV infection among drug injectors in New York City has been reported as hovering around 60% for several years. In San Francisco, a city that has a comparable rate of HIV infection to New York City among male homosexuals, the seroprevalence rate among intravenous drug users has been consistently reported as approximately 15%. One possible explanation for the large difference in seroprevalence rates could be the nature of shooting galleries used for drug injection in each city (Watters, 1989; Des Jarlais, & Friedman, 1990). Needles used for injecting in commercial galleries have been shown to be especially virulent (Chitwood, McCoy, Inciardi et al., 1990). Moreover, some of the same sociodemographic characteristics associated with increased rates of infection among samples of drug injectors have also been shown to be associated with increased use by addicts of commercial shooting galleries (Celentano, Vlahov, Cohn et al., 1991). Whereas shooting galleries in New York City are commercial establishments attracting large numbers of drug injectors, a shooting gallery in San Francisco is a noncommercial affair organized around small friendship groups (Murphy, & Waldorf, 1991). The presence and use of commercial shooting galleries may indeed account for the variation in seroprevalence rates among drug injectors in New York City and San Francisco.

Although the context of drug injection as an explanation of varying seroprevalence rates among samples of intravenous drug users does increase our understanding, it may lack the qualities of a satisfactory explanation of varying HIV infection rates for two reasons. First, despite variations in the context of drug use, HIV infection among geographically distinct populations of intravenous drug users should approach uniformity over time without effective prevention measures or other significant intervening variables. Second, the context of drug injection as an explanation discounts sexual behaviors as mechanisms of viral transmission. Although the relative effects of drug (i.e., needle) use and sexual behaviors have not yet been disentangled, without specific contrary evidence, sexual transmission of the virus among injection drug users must be taken into account in any explanation of varying seroprevalence rates.

Not only is it necessary to understand the context, the behaviors, and conditions of intravenous drug use in explaining the rates of HIV infection among geographically distinct populations, it is also necessary to understand with whom and how injectors connect or are linked to one another. Analysis of the social network structures of intravenous drug users may provide a more complete explanation of varying seroprevalence rates. A social network is the sum of linkages among people in a defined population (Klovdahl, 1985). Social networks are aggregates of personal networks; the sum of connections or linkages between individuals. Linkages between individuals are, of course, not all the same. Interpersonal links vary along a number of relevant factors: length of interaction and frequency of contact, number of contacts, heterogeneity of contacts, and strength of emotional ties (Auslander, & Litwen; Granovetter, 1973; Marsden, 1987; Pilisuk, & Froland, 1978; Saulnier, & Rowland, 1975). The sum of variations in individual linkages produces patterns of social network structures which have a strong effect on the transmission of communicable diseases. "[T]he structure of a network has consequences for its individual members and for the [social] network as a whole over and above effects of characteristics and behavior of the individuals involved" (Klovdahl, 1985, p. 1204).

The purpose of this paper is to present data from an ethnographic investigation of intravenous drug users' social network structures in Houston, Texas. Social networks are defined as the aggregate of drug injection or sexual interpersonal connections or links among illicit drug injectors residing in two targeted communities. Data were collected at the level of personal networks. From the typologies which emerged characterizing personal network structures, a model of the social network structure was developed.

METHODS

Data for this study were collected between July, 1991 and January, 1992 from a purposive sample of intravenous drug users (Johnson, 1990). Participants in the ethnographic study were selected from a larger sample of drug injectors residing in two targeted geographic areas in Houston recruited to participate in a quantitative investigation of intravenous drug use and HIV risk behaviors. Participants in the quantitative study were recruited based on place of residence. Geographic areas of the city were selected and targeted for recruitment as the result of an assessment of rates of drug related crimes, arrests for prostitution, and calls to emergency medical services for drug overdoses. Trained outreach workers went into the target areas to recruit participants by frequenting copping areas identified by ethnographic mapping and through personal contacts with drug injectors. Intravenous drug users successfully recruited to participate in the quantitative study were requested to refer friends and acquaintances who also injected drugs (Watters, & Biernacki, 1989; Johnson, 1990). Requirements for participation in the study were evidence of recent drug injection, confirmed by puncture wounds or marks on the skin, reported drug injection in the 30 days before the study, and no history of enrollment in drug treatment during the 30 days prior to participation. Study participants were also required to be 18 years of age or older, reside within the boundaries of the targeted areas, provide sufficient information for relocation, and to have signed an informed consent.

Intravenous drug users who appeared to be knowledgeable about drug use scenes in their neighborhoods were referred by outreach workers for inclusion in this study. Information provided about an individual by an outreach worker and data collected for relocation, which included the number of injectors who would know the whereabouts of the individual, also were assessed. A list of likely candidates for inclusion in this study was compiled. Those who appeared to be most knowledgeable about drug injection activities within the targeted areas were recontacted by outreach workers and asked to participate in an interview about how intravenous drug users organized their daily drug use activities. Data were collected from 39 men, 7 women, 26 African-Americans, 6 Hispanics, and 14 Caucasian injectors. The relative proportions of men to women and among racial/ethnic groups were chosen to reflect the composition of the drug injecting population residing in the targeted geographic areas.

Data were collected using in-depth, guided conversational interviews (Patton, 1990). Two formats were selected for interviewing. Thirty-two respondents were interviewed in small groups. A targeted respondent was invited to bring his/her close drug using friends and associates with him to the interview. Fourteen interviews were conducted with only the targeted individual. All interviews were conducted in a private setting by a trained researcher. Although the interviewer had a predetermined set of open-ended questions covering everyday activities, including the number and activities of a respondent's network members, the interviewer was free to pursue topics introduced by the respondent which the interviewer felt provided useful information. The focus of the guided interviews were the "everyday" activities and interactions of study participants.To avoid interviewer selective recall, interviews were recorded by notes and audio tape recordings. All interviews were assessed for topics and typologies to generate questions to be included in subsequent interviews. Study participants were compensated for their time.

Interviews were transcribed verbatim onto computer templates for analysis. The data were analyzed for typologies which emerged from the data about injectors' everyday interactions and activities. These in turn were assessed for the number and frequency of interpersonal links, heterogeneity of links, composition of interpersonal links, and strength of emotional links among individuals related to either injected drug use or sexual activities (Auslander, & Litwin, 1987; Marsden, 1987; Pilisuk, & Forland, 1978; Reiss, 1990; Saulnier, & Rowland, 1985). The time frame used for reference was during the course of a normal day. The number and duration of drug use interpersonal links was defined as the number of people with whom an injector interacted and how frequently the interactions were likely to occur. Heterogeneity was defined as the gender, age, and racial diversity of drug using persons with whom an injector interacted. Composition of links was defined as the category of individuals, such as relative, friend, acquaintance, with whom a drug injector interacted during the course of a normal day. The strength of emotional links was defined as the intensity of emotional ties between linked individuals. Analysis of network characteristics was limited to drug use or sexual interpersonal links. Collectively, these links were characterized as those interpersonal interactions which could potentially transmit HIV.

Data were first assessed for typologies of personal drug use linkages within the targeted communities (Miles, & Huberman, 1984). Typologies which were constructed for the factors: number and frequency, heterogeneity, composition, and strength of emotional links within personal drug use networks, were used to conceptually derive patterns of strong and weak links among individuals (Granovetter, 1973). A composite of strong and weak network linkages was used to develop a model of the social network structure of intravenous drug use within the city.

DRUG INJECTION PERSON NETWORKS

Number of Interpersonal Linkages and Frequency of Interactions

The number of everyday links between drug injectors involving drug use or sexual activities tend to be relatively small. The majority of sexual links occur between people who are "regular," long-term sexual partners. Respondents reported regularly injecting or sharing drugs with one to five other users with whom they had injected for a number of years. The most commonly reported number of drug users regularly injecting together was three. The answers provided by Elroy and Robert were typical of injectors describing their everyday drug use interactions.

> Interviewer: So how many people do you shoot drugs with and still stay with?
>
> Elroy: Oh, very few. Very, very few.
>
> Interviewer: About how many?
>
> Elroy: About two.
>
> Robert: Two or three, yeah.

Although injectors said that they regularly shared drugs, injected or had sex with a relatively small number of other users with whom they had been involved for a long time, respondents did report being in contact with a large number of other drug users on an average day. Most often these contacts were reported as activities related to purchasing drugs or activities of lifestyle, such as hanging out. Communication was the most commonly reported activity. News of drug supplies, police activities, and the activities of other users were reported as important topics of conversation. For example, the comments of one group of two White women and one White man illustrates the importance of communication as an activity:

> Jim: Well, you know, if somebody is getting busted, that means somebody else is going to get it.
>
> Rochelle: A lot of other people are worried they will.
>
> Jim: Usually when they make a bust, they're not going to make just one. Usually when they come in an area, they want to get something. Get somewhere. So you let [other injectors] know what's going on.
>
> Interviewer: So it's not just protection for your friends?

Jim: It's like the, what they call 'em there, the Houston tactical team. You know, if they're involved, something is going on.

Injectors maintain a number of interpersonal communication links. Out of these linkages, opportunities for drug injection or sexual activities sometimes occur.

Infrequently, contacts among users who are not regular drug injecting partners do result in drug injection episodes. These episodes are considered by injectors to be out of the ordinary and not a part of daily drug injection activity. Drug injection with individuals other than regular partners are not planned, but the result of chance. Users refer to these random opportunities for drug use as "come and go's." An Hispanic male injector depicted occasions for drug injection with other users that would just "pop up":

Hey, _____ , you got five dollars, let's go get a fifty-fifty, or a half-n-half. Let me use your rig. Hey, _____ , can I use your room. Things like that.

The opportunity for drug use is the basis for the link among drug injecting acquaintances and the connection usually lasts no longer than the actual drug injection scene. Besides an unforeseen chance to get high, unplanned opportunities for sex also emerge from the daily interactions with other drug users. A number of male injectors reported occasions when an unexpected windfall of money and the presence of female crack users looking for drugs provided an occasion for a sexual interlude. A 41-year-old African-American man reported:

If you want some sex, you just get some crack. There are about a hundred rock stars out there. You want her, you know she smokes crack and you want her, just get you some crack. She'll do whatever you want her to do. It don't matter. You get her as long as you want.

Although the number of women, especially crack users, willing to trade sex for drugs was reported as high, the number and frequency of sexual encounters among drug injecting men and women trading sex for crack was not an everyday occurrence.

Most drug injectors do not rely on casual relationships as the basis of their drug injection lifestyles. However, two types of individuals were reported as fulfilling roles within the community of injectors which are based on building and maintaining a number of casual relationships. Runners typically develop relationships with several drug dealers and users as the method used for earning a living or supporting their drug using habit. A runner will buy drugs for other injectors and, as payment, receive a portion of the drugs either for personal use or for resale. Runners cultivate relationships with other injectors who they may not know well and interact with infrequently. As Calbern, a 40-year-old African-American male runner, explained:

Interviewer: How do you know everybody?

Calbern: 'Cause I be on the corner of the drugs every day. I be up there every day. I sell drugs if I can get a hold of some.

Interviewer: Are you a dealer?

Calbern: Nah, man. If I can get enough money to where I can buy enough quantity to flip it up and get my money back so I can make me some money, I do.

Interviewer: [Y]ou are not a drug dealer?

Calbern: I know what a drug dealer is. I know the dealer to call. All I got to do is beep him. I call him right now and he come up here . . . I might shoot four or five times a day and that come out to fifty or sixty people. It all depends on who I run into and who got the money. You ain't got no money, I ain't finnin' to get you nothin.'

A second type of injector who cultivates and maintains a number of casual relationships with other injectors is a houseman. A houseman is a man or woman who provides his(her) apartment or house as a safe place for users to inject and, in return, receives drugs or money as a fee. Housemen do not sell drugs, but may sell needles besides providing a place for injection.

Interviewer: Where were you at?

Wiesel: Over there off Y_____.

Interviewer: Was it a house or apartment?
Slim: Yeah, like an opium den.

Bruce: Yeah, you go in and you shoot.

Slim: They got rigs . . . It's a neighborhood thing. Everybody know'd everybody goin' in. You know the dude that got the house. You say, "Hey man, I got to do this here. I need to shoot this here up."

Wiesel: He get you a syringe.

Slim: He get you the water and you go over there and shoot the stuff up.

Interviewer: What did the guy get for letting you use his house to inject?

Slim: Oh, we give him five units.

Bruce: Sometimes we give 'im one dollar or two dollars.

Slim: It depend on if he a real user like us. That dollar or two, we can keep that. We just have to give him some of the medicine.

Occasionally, housemen may provide a room for a fee in which users can have sex. But, this is a far less common activity than selling space where drugs can be injected. Like runners, housemen cultivate casual relationships with a number of drug injectors. Occasionally, the roles of runner and houseman will be played by a single individual. This person provides a location in which drugs can be injected and will interact with a dealer to purchase drugs.

Heterogeneity of Interpersonal Linkages

Everyday interactions between drug injectors and other drug users tend to be among individuals who are homogeneous in terms of age, gender, education, and ethnic characteristics. Injectors, as a group, reported interacting and using drugs with others who were like themselves. The most frequent grouping of long-term injection partners was among men. Women were on the periphery of these relationships, rarely participating in drug injection activities. Two white male injectors reported:

> Scott: There're very few girls in our neighborhood.

> Cajun: That's true. But, like the other reason, if you bring a girl in there to shoot dope it's because you want to fuck her. That's the point. She's trying to get high. But the rule is, if you give her some dope, she's got to give you some pussy.

Except for couples, which are predominantly of mixed gender, everyday drug use relationships tend to be formed among men.

If a woman is present in a drug injection group of more than two persons, she is most likely the sexual partner of one of the male members and the only female member in the group. As well, drug injectors rarely conduct everyday drug use activities with injectors of another ethnic or racial group. African-Americans tend to limit their drug injection relationships to other African-Americans. Hispanics rarely interact with non-Hispanics.

> Interviewer: Do you guys ever shoot up or hang out with White guys or Hispanic guys?

> Wiesel: Me, myself? I don't.

> Slim: Mostly I drink methadone with 'em. That's right. At the VA.

> Bruce: Mostly I don't. I had one White partner. Now we was in the penitentiary together. We used to mess around, but he went to California.

Drug using links between members of different racial groups are rare. On occasions when injectors of different racial groups do interact, it is usually Caucasians and African-Americans or Caucasians and Hispanics who inject together as the consequence of unplanned opportunities for injecting.

Casual drug use relationships also tend to be homogeneous with regard to race/ethnicity and gender. A partial explanation for the racial/ethnic homogeneity of drug injection linkages in Houston is geographic territory. Injectors' territories are areas of the city bounded by interstate highways, bayous, or other boundaries. As a consequence of history, most territories within the city are racially segregated. Drug injectors tend to live out their lives in the area of the city where they spent their childhoods. The injectors interviewed reported preferring the familiarity and safety of their own areas, where people are known and relationships are predictable. As one Hispanic male drug injector reported:

> These is my stompin' grounds. Why should I go over there, when the drugs are over here?

The police also act to encourage injectors to restrict their activities to home territories. Police officers are most likely to stop and question individuals who do not seem to fit their surroundings. Drug users run a greater risk of being questioned by the police if they are in a territory of differing racial characteristics. Casual drug use links tend to be among men because of the mileau in which the random opportunities for drug use occur. Most male drug injectors will hangout on a favorite street corner or frequent a small number of business establishments. These are male environments which women do not ordinarily frequent. Women who are found on the streets or in male dominated business establishments tend to be there for the purposes of exchanging sex for money.

Everyday and casual interpersonal drug injection activities are also restricted by drug of choice. The most apparent dichotomy which emerges is between drug injectors and crack cocaine smokers. Injectors characterize crack smokers as "bad" people, and blame crack smokers for increasing drug related violence and the social decline of their neighborhoods. Under most circumstances, intravenous drug users will avoid crack smokers. Clarence, an African-American man, reported his impression of crack smokers:

> This is a lot different from the way things was before. The difference is dope ain't as good and there are so many people with this rock stuff. Man, people just don't have the class they used to have. They gone to the dogs. They have no morals. They don't care. They get it any way they can do it. Man, they got them little girls who will turn a flip for you for just a hit. Violence, these people will stab you in the back for ten dollars.

It's the crack users. They're the ones that be violent out there. These IV users, there're a few who are violent, but not like these crack heads.

Clarence's comments were typical of most of the injectors.

However, some male drug injectors will take advantage of an opportunity for sex with female crack smokers needing money or drugs. Males reported buying crack and parceling it out a little at a time to female crack addicts in exchange for an evening of sex:

Robin: That rock! The only time I mess with rock is with these girls that don't want to do nothin' but rock. And, she gotta, you know, do somethin' before I give her the first rock. Hey, I'm sorry. "Bitch, you got to suck my dick while I'm hittin' on this." Or . . .

John: That's the way it goes.

Robin: Hey, I'm sorry, but that's the only way I'll mess with it.

John: "Hey, come over here. Why don't you knock down on this thing here while I do a hit?" Hey, that's my favorite shot.

Robin: Shit. That's my shot.

Another linkage between drug injectors and crack smokers are a small number of individuals who both inject and smoke crack. Usually these individuals have a preferred method of ingestion and will maintain the most numerous and strongest drug use relationships with others who ingest in the preferred manner. Yet, some interpersonal linkages will be fostered with those who ingest in the less preferred way.

Composition of Interpersonal Linkages

The composition of interpersonal linkages varies depending on whether or not drug injection is with regular or casual injection partners. The composition of linkages which emerged from the interviews related to everyday drug use and sharing activities were based upon sexual, familial, or shared histories. Sexual partners or "couples" form drug using linkages directly related to their sexual intimacy. Links with other drug injectors by couples tend to be infrequent. Interactions between couples and other drug users which do occur are usually those necessary to purchase drugs. For example, one couple reported:

> Norma: Well, if you're talking about any kind of sex, drugs, or whatever, nothing. This is my only sex partner and my only partner I do drugs with. Today, any day, whatever.
>
> Joe: Same thing with me.
>
> Interviewer: Do you and him ever do drugs with other people?
>
> Norma: No.
>
> Joe: We really don't. Like when we go somewhere, we're at somebody's house, we go by ourselves. We go to a room.
>
> Norma: We go to, like, our own room. We like to be alone because we trip on each other.

Family relationships also form the basis of frequent drug use linkages. Most often brothers, sisters, or cousins form close attachments among themselves for the purpose of drug injection. One group's comments illustrate family members as preferred regular drug injection partners:

> June: See, some of them you can't trust. You can't give nobody your money and tell them to go buy you [some dope]. They might not come back. They keep going.
>
> John: There's nobody out there I trust really.
>
> Interviewer: But, you said you trust each other.
>
> John: Family.
>
> June: I give them my money and they're going to come back with mine.

A third pattern of composition among regular drug injecting partners is based on a shared history, including the use of drugs. A number of respondents reported regularly injecting drugs with individuals they knew as children or with whom they attended high school. At minimum, users reported knowledge of a regular shooting partner from a member of the partner's family or others in the neighborhood prior to forming a long term drug injection relationship. In the following example, John and June are cousins, Mason is not related:

> June: We grow'd up together in the same neighborhood. I know him for years. People in his family. Well, one of his brothers had a kid by one of my stepsisters. We know each other.

> Mason: We like kin to each other.

> John: We smokes together. I been around when he [Mason] shoot up. I used to shoot dope, too. She's the oldest one. But, she done see us come up. We're about six, seven years younger than her, but she's seen us come up.

Less frequently, jail or prison were mentioned as the shared history between individuals who regularly injected together.

The composition of linkages during less frequently occurring opportunistic occasions for drug use were less restrictive, but still limited. Users reported that they would only take advantage of an opportunity for drug injection if the other participants were known from the home territory. Most injectors who were interviewed reported that drugs were never shared when an unknown person was a member of the opportunistic drug use group. Strangers were only admitted to drug use activities when an injector who was known could vouch for a stranger's integrity. The report of this group was typical:

> Interviewer: If somebody new comes in, how do they get in with you?

> Robert: They get in from somebody else that you know or somebody that's close to you. Like, "man, this is Doug. This, that, or the other."

Rob: That we know, he alright.

Elroy: But, they still gonna have to . . .

Rob: But, you still, yourself, gonna keep a kinda high arm.
Robert: That's alright for that particular night with me. But, he ever come back . . .

Rob: Without him . . .

Robert: Yeah, without him, I'm gonna be impersonal. "No, no, don't you never, huh, uh. I don't never."
"But, I was with so and so."
"Well, where is he? When you get back with him, come back and see me. I know who you talkin' about, but I don't know you."

Elroy: That's right.

Users reported categorically excluding certain types of people from their opportunistic drug using activities. People who were known to act crazy or become violent, injectors who routinely could not contribute to purchasing drugs or were thought to have stolen from other users, suspected police informants, or adolescents were mentioned as the types of individuals routinely excluded. As well, injectors who were suspected of being HIV positive or having AIDS were excluded from opportunistic injection activities.

Opportunistic drug use situations are not always limited solely to drug users or drug use activities. Occasionally the composition of the group includes women, usually crack users, who have been recruited for sex. Sex is a medium of exchange through which women can get drugs, although the exchange may not be viewed as prostitution. As in other situations where the social expectation is that the male provide a dinner and an evening's entertainment before romance, the social expectation is that if a woman goes with a man to "party," the man provides the drugs. As Clarence, an African-American man reported:

If I see one [a woman] I like . . . you know. I get me a room and I buy me some drugs. I like to stay in there and spend a thousand dollars. But once you leave that room, she's gonna have another. I might be broke, but she's gonna be broke, too.

A woman's entry into opportunistic drug using groups is not as rigorous as that for injectors. A woman's willingness to "party" is usually sufficient criteria.

Strength of Emotional Linkages

The strongest emotional linkages among intravenous users occur between members of a regular drug using group. Usually intimacy is a function of time and exchanges. Emotional linkages are strongest between drug using partners who have shared drugs for many years. Regular drug using partners stated that their expectations were that partners "watch each other's backs."

Interviewer: So you guys trust each other.

John: Oh yeah.

Robin: I know he gonna watch my back and I'm gonna watch his,

John: Nothin' gonna happen to us. This man could o.d.

Robin: I know I'm alright. That's why I told the guy who asked, "Hey, do you shoot by yourself?" I said, "I ain't gonna shoot by myself."

Couples, as well, are expected to watch "each other's backs," but are also expected to "keep each other from going down." "Going down" was described as allowing drug use to get out of control to the point where it would threaten the relationship.

A particularly important emotional link between regular injection partners was characterized by those interviewed as trust. Trust is invested in another individual only after a slow and difficult process of building and maintaining a relationship. Trust can be bestowed at different levels and, of course, withdrawn. Trust implies that drugs and the resources necessary to buy drugs will be shared. The amount of drugs or money shared among regular partners need not be equal, but something must be contributed. Having a small number of others who can be trusted has survival advantages. Trusted partners can act as lookouts for the police or trouble, comfort one another during bad drug reactions, or provide first aid in case of an overdose. An aspect of trust, which is not part of a usual definition, includes trusting another with one's high:

Interviewer: Why would somebody else blow your high?

John: They go to aggravate you, so you not enjoy it.

Rob: See some people go through changes.

John: Some people have a different rationale, a different personality.

Rob: See, it [cocaine] don't do 'em all the same. See.

John: Some dope not made for . . .

Rob: Everybody. But, they do it.

John: But, they can't handle it. They may not act like that otherwise.

Injectors use drugs to experience the pleasure produced by the high. Injectors who become violent, act belligerent, cannot control their paranoia, or act "crazy," interfere with the pleasure of the drug using experience and, therefore, cannot be trusted not to interfere with one's high.

In lieu of emotional linkages, links between drug users who are casual acquaintances function according to explicit and implicit expectations attached to the roles played. The expectations of drug injectors are referred to as "the rules." For example, when users pool money to buy drugs, the order in which drugs are injected is determined by how much money was contributed, who took the risks of buying, and who is supplying a place where the drugs can be injected. An individual who buys the drugs for an injection scene has the right to inject first. A houseman has the prerogative of receiving a taste of the drug because he(she) has provided a safe place for injecting. A runner has the right to a high rank in the injection order because he(she) has taken the risks associated with purchasing the drugs. An individual who has not made a contribution toward either purchasing or providing for the shared drug injection experience, a "hanger-on," is entitled to nothing and must depend on the altruistic inclinations of those who have contributed. The rules are characterized by users as respect. To violate the rules means to violate the "respect" owed another. Not all rules are derived from the economics of drug purchasing. Some of "the rules" are similar to expectations among more intimate drug users. For example, the rule that users respect each other's high by not acting "neurotic" is very similar to the expectations of trusting another with one's high among intimates.

SOCIAL NETWORK STRUCTURES: STRONG AND WEAK LINKS

The typologies of interpersonal injection and sexual linkages which emerged along the factors of number and duration, heterogeneity, composition, and strength of emotional bonds can be used to identify linkage as strong or weak (Granovetter, 1973). Generally, strong interpersonal links are those which are frequent over a long period of time, homogeneous, limited to a relatively small group of people, and exhibit strong emotional bonds among group members. Weak interpersonal links are those which are infrequent and last a short duration, heterogeneous, involve a relatively large number of persons having varied relationships, and exhibit weak emotional bonds among the people involved in the interaction. The data presented above suggest that most drug injectors in Houston have strong and weak links to other drug injectors and sexual partners. However, the largest proportion of drug injection or sexual activities occurs among people who are strongly linked. A small number of injectors, for example couples, will exhibit few, if any, weak drug injection or sexual links to others within their communities. As well, a small number, such as drug runners or housemen, will have a large number of weak drug injection links and may have no strong links to other injectors. Characterizing linkages as strong or weak allows a hypothetical model of the structure of intravenous drug injectors' social network to be constructed. The aggregate of personal drug injection or sexual links produces a model of the social network structure related to drug injection and sexual activities as shown in Figure 1.

Figure 1 shows that the largest number of drug injectors represented are strongly linked to between one and four other drug injectors. Consistent with our interview data, the largest number of injectors are strongly bonded with two other intravenous users making a drug injection clique. Drug injection or sexual activities which occur outside the small cliques of drug injectors are ordinarily the result of unexpected opportunities for drug use, sexual activities, or both. Thus, unexpected drug injection or sexual activities are characterized by weak interpersonal links between cliques. As was reported in the interviews, a small number of cliques, represented in the figure by drug injectors 16 and 17, do not interact with other

FIGURE 1

MODEL DRUG INJECTION AND SEXUAL SOCIAL
NETWORK STRUCTURE IN HOUSTON, TEXAS

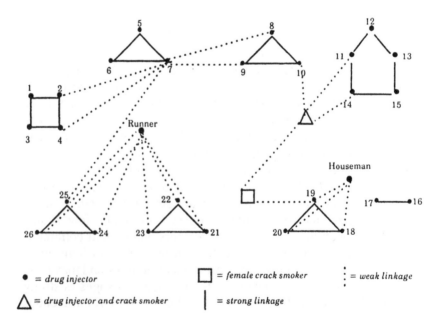

injectors either to share drugs or for sex. As well, a small number of individuals cultivate only weak links with other injectors. In the figure, these individuals are represented by the intravenous users labeled "runner" and "houseman." Other types of individuals were also mentioned in the interviews as not strongly linked to any drug injection clique. Female crack smokers and individuals who use both injected drugs and crack, but who prefer crack, will take advantage of opportunistic occasions to share injected drugs or, in the case of female crack smokers, exchange sex for crack. Most drug injection and sexual activity among intravenous drug users in Houston occurs within strongly linked cliques.

Houston is composed of several well bounded geographic areas as a result of historical influences and distance. As shown in Figure 2, it can be expected that the city will contain a number of intravenous drug using social networks bounded by geography and race/ethnicity. Injectors of different racial groups rarely interact with one another. Interaction among social networks which do take place are infrequent. Links between social networks are most likely to occur between members of the same racial/ethnic group or between African-Americans and Caucasians or Hispanics and Caucasians. Injectors simply prefer the familiarity and routine of their home areas. A factor which may encourage the relative isolation of drug injection social networks is distance. Like many American cities in the west, Houston is a sprawling metropolis lacking a well developed mass transit system. Trips between areas are time consuming and, if an injector does not have a car or money for alternative transportation, travel is hard on the feet. For many users, it is just easier to stay on home turf. The result of these patterns of behavior is a number of isolated drug using social networks bounded by area and racial/ethnic characteristics. Connections which occur between the social networks are weak.

DISCUSSION

This study presented ethnographic data on the composition of personal drug injection networks in Houston, Texas. The personal linkages among drug injectors were assessed for variation on the

FIGURE 2

INTRAVENOUS DRUG USE SOCIAL
NETWORK STRUCTURES IN HOUSTON

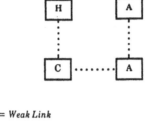

A = African-American

C = Caucasian   ⋮ = Weak Link

H = Hispanic

factors number and duration, heterogeneity, composition, and emotional intensity of links among intravenous drug injectors. From an analysis of these factors, a pattern of strong and weak interpersonal links among injectors emerged. The largest portion of drug injecting and sexual contacts among injectors occur among individuals who are strongly linked. Drug use and sexual contacts involving weak links are less frequent and appear to be random events. The concepts of strong and weak links informed an attempt to model a drug injectors' social network structure. The structure represents a number of small drug injecting cliques connected to one another in the social network by weak links. This structure characterizes drug injectors in Houston as isolated by geographic territory and racial/ethnic characteristics. The result being a number of relatively isolated drug injecting social networks coexisting within the city.

The significance of the social network structures of intravenous drug users in understanding rates of HIV infection among intravenous drug users is in understanding the significance of weak drug injection and sexual links among injectors and others within a community. Small groups of people or cliques are linked to one another through weak links. For example, flow of information, job mobility, and adoption of innovation have been shown to be related to the number of weak links within a social network structure (Granovetter, 1973). Where groups or cliques do not have weak links, they are isolated. Removing or adding weak links among cliques substantially alters the structure of a social network. The transmission of HIV is dependent on interpersonal behaviors. Therefore, how people within a social network structure are linked is key to understanding the spread of the virus within a population. If groups of intravenous drug users do not have weak links to other groups of drug injectors, such as injectors 16 and 17 in Figure 1, the chances of a member of a group becoming infected are, no matter how "high risk" their behavior, remote. Groups of injectors who have a number of weak links to other groups of injectors run a much greater risk of infection, even if they infrequently engage in "high risk" behaviors. For example, injector 1 in Figure 1 is not directly linked to any other injector outside his personal clique. However, because injector 1's clique members, injectors 2 and 4, are weakly linked to injector 7, injector 1 is indirectly connected to every other individual depicted in Figure 1, except injectors 17 and 16. The implications for injector 1 are that, even if he does not participate in risky behaviors outside his clique, if any other injector to whom he is indirectly linked becomes HIV infected, injector 1 has a high probability of becoming infected.

Modeling the social network structures of intravenous drug injectors can substantially help explain the variation in HIV infection rates among populations of injectors throughout the United States. It can be hypothesized that low seroprevalence populations will either have a limited number of weak links among groups of injectors residing in the area and/or few weak linkages to drug injectors in other, higher seroprevalence areas. The data presented by Battjes, Pickens, and Amsel (1989) concerning the introduction of HIV into a population of drug injectors would not be inconsistent with this hypothesis. An analysis of weak links among groups of injectors residing within a locality can also help explain varying HIV infection rates among different populations within the local area. For example, in Houston, infection rates vary by race and gender. Among men, African-American intravenous drug users have an approximate infection rate of 10%, Caucasians 7%, and Hispanics 4% (Williams, 1990). Men have a higher HIV infection rate than women. Preliminary analysis of ethnographic data suggests that Hispanics and women in Houston are far more likely to restrict drug injection and sexual activities to others with whom they are strongly linked. African-American and Caucasian men are more likely to be members of drug injection cliques that are weakly linked to a number of other drug injecting groups. Female drug injectors and Hispanics would be expected to have lower seroprevalence rates because of their relative lack of weak links to other injectors. An analysis of weak links can also help predict the future course of the epidemic. For example, using Figure 1 as a method of prediction, it would be expected that crack smokers in Houston will experience an expanding HIV infection rate. Further, it can be predicted that the most likely vector for transmission of the virus into the crack-smoking population will be women who trade sex to intravenous drug users for crack or crack smokers who also inject. Early analysis of seroprevalence data on crack smokers in Houston provides some support for this hypothesis (Williams, 1992). Analysis of a sample of drug injectors and crack smokers has found that female crack smokers had a seroprevalence rate roughly equivalent to drug injecting men and higher than drug injecting women.

Focusing research on the structure of intravenous drug use social networks and especially on weak links among cliques of drug injectors may be useful in designing HIV prevention strategies. As was related here, the emotional bonds among drug injection clique members are very strong. The bonds center around a social value of trust which may govern needle sharing and sexual behaviors. Modification of needle sharing or sexual behaviors within cliques is likely to be extremely difficult. Refusing to share a needle, the use of bleach, or the wearing of a condom may involve a violation of trust, which for regular drug sharing or sexual partners may have more significance than the risk of HIV infection (see Grund, Kaplan, & Adriaans, 1991; van den Hock, van Haastrecht, & Coutinho, 1992). It may be far more beneficial to focus prevention efforts on modifying or reducing weak link drug injection and sexual behaviors. Weak link behaviors are less likely to involve strong emotional ties among injectors and are already governed by a set of rules. Modifying the "rules" to include avoidance of causal drug use or sexual encounters or practicing prevention behaviors may hold promise.

Of course, this study is limited by the lack of a random sample from which findings could be generalized. As well, to fully model the social network structure of drug injectors in Houston, a study capable of quantitatively measuring the links within and between groups of intravenous drug injectors needs to be conducted. Yet, the findings of this study do suggest that understanding the social network structures of intravenous drug injectors would significantly contribute to our understanding of the epidemiology of HIV infection among drug injectors and, perhaps, lead to the development of more effective disease prevention measures.

REFERENCES

Alperin S. and R. Needle (1991). Social network analysis: An approach for understanding IV drug users in Community-Based AIDS Prevention: Studies of Intravenous Drug Users and Their Sexual Partners. Rockville, MD: U.S. Department of Health and Human Services.

Auslander G. and H. Litwin (1987). The parameters of network intervention: A social work application. Social Service Review 61: 305-318.

Battjes R., R. Pickens and Z. Amsel (1989). Introduction of HIV infection among intravenous drug abusers in low prevalence areas. Journal of Acquired Immune Deficiency Syndromes 2: 533-539.

Celentano D., D. Vlahov, S. Cohn, Anthony, Solomon, and Nelson (1991). Risk factors for shooting gallery use and cessation among intravenous drug users. American Journal of Public Health 81: 1291-1295.

Chitwood D., C. McCoy, J. Inciardi, D. McBride, M. Comerford, E. Trapido E., H. McCoy, J. Page, J. Griffin, M. Fletcher, and Ashman M. (1990). HIV Seropositivity of needles from shooting galleries in south Florida. American Journal of Public Health 80: 150-152.

Des Jarlais D. and S. Friedman (1990). Shooting galleries and AIDS: Infection probabilities and 'tough' policies. American Journal of Public Health 80: 142-144.

Des Jarlais D., S. Friedman, and C. Casriel (1990). Target groups for preventing AIDS among intravenous drug users: 2. The "hard" data studies. Journal of Consulting and Clinical Psychology 58: 50-56.

Granovetter M. (1973). The strength of weak ties. American Journal of Sociology 78: 1360-1380.

Grund J., C. Kaplan, and N. Adriaans (1991). Needle sharing in the Netherlands: An ethnographic analysis. American Journal of Public Health 81: 1602-1607.

van den Hoek J., H. van Haastrecht, and R. Coutinho (1992). Little change in sexual behavior in injecting drug users in Amsterdam. Journal of Acquired Immune Deficiency Syndromes 5: 518-522.

Hummond N. and P. Doreian (1990). Computational methods for social network analysis. Social Networks 12: 270-285.

Johnson J.C. (1990). Selecting Ethnographic Informants. Newberry Park, CA: Sage Publications.

Klovdahl A. (1985). Social networks and the spread of infectious diseases: The AIDS example. Social Science Medicine 21: 1203-1216.

Marsden P. (1987). Core discussion networks of Americans. American Sociological Review 52: 122-131.

Miles M. and A. Huberman (1984). Qualitative Data Analysis: A Source Book of New Methods. Newbury Park, CA: Sage Publications.

Murphy S. and D. Waldorf (1991). Kickin' down to the street doc: Shooting galleries in the San Francisco Bay area. Contemporary Drug Problems Spring: 9-29.

Patton M. (1990). Qualitative Evaluation and Research Methods. Newbury Park, CA: Sage Publications.

Pilisuk M. and C. Froland (1978). Kinship, social networks, social support and health. Social Science and Medicine 12B: 273-280.

Reis H. (1990). The role of intimacy in interpersonal relations. Journal of Social and Clinical Psychology 9: 15-30.

Saulnier K. and C. Rowland (1985). Missing links: An empirical investigation of network variables in high-risk families. Family Relations 34: 557-560.

Siegal H., R. Carlson, R. Falck, L. Li, M. Forney, R. Rapp, K. Baumgartner, W. Meyers, M. Nelson (1991). HIV infection and risk behaviors among intravenous drug users in low seroprevalence areas in the midwest. American Journal of Public Health 81: 1642-1644.

Watters J. (1988). Meaning and context: The social facts of intravenous drug use and HIV transmission in the inner city. Journal of Psychoactive Drugs 20: 173-177.

Watters J. (1989). Observations on the importance of social context in HIV transmission among intravenous drug users. Journal of Drug Issues 19: 9-26.

Williams M. (1990). HIV seroprevalence among male IVDUs in Houston, Texas. American Journal of Public Health 80: 1507-1509.

Williams M. (1992). Semiannual report to the National Institute on Drug Abuse. Unpublished data.

Woodhouse D., J. Patterat, A. Klovdahl, W. Darrow, S. Muth, and J. Muth (1990). Social networks in the transmission of HIV infection. Sixth Annual Conference on AIDS, San Francisco, CA.

Copping Areas as Sampling and Recruitment Sites for Out-of-Treatment Crack and Injection Drug Users

Rafaela R. Robles, EdD
Héctor M. Colón, MA
Daniel H. Freeman, PhD

SUMMARY. Monitoring behaviors and serostatus of drug addicts requires the recruitment and assessment of successive samples of the not-in-treatment population. Sampling of street addicts presents a number of difficult methodological problems. This paper describes the strategies used to implement random sampling strategies in the recruitment of out-of-treatment crack and injection drug users in the

Rafaela R. Robles is affiliated with the Center for Sociomedical Research, School of Public Health, Medical Sciences Campus, University of Puerto Rico and Research Institute, Puerto Rico Department of Anti Addiction Services, San Juan, PR. Héctor M. Colón is affiliated with the Research Institute, Puerto Rico Department of Anti Addiction Services, San Juan, PR. Daniel H. Freeman is affiliated with the Office of Biostatistics, University of Texas Medical Branch, Galveston, TX.

Please address correspondence to: Research Institute, Puerto Rico Department of Anti Addiction Services, P.O. Box 21414, Rio Piedras Station, Rio Piedras, PR 00928-1414.

[Haworth co-indexing entry note]: "Copping Areas as Sampling and Recruitment Sites for Out-of-Treatment Crack and Injection Drug Users." Robles, Rafaela R., Héctor M. Colón, and Daniel H. Freeman. Co-published simultaneously in *Drugs & Society* (The Haworth Press, Inc.) Vol. 7, No. 3/4, 1993, pp. 91-105; and: *AIDS and Community-Based Drug Intervention Programs: Evaluation and Outreach* (ed: Dennis G. Fisher, and Richard Needle), The Haworth Press, Inc., 1993, pp. 91-105. Multiple copies of this article/chapter may be purchased from The Haworth Document Delivery Center [1-800-3-HAWORTH; 9:00 a.m. - 5:00 p.m. (EST)].

Copyright © 1993 by Taylor & Francis

San Juan Metropolitan Area. A three-stage sampling procedure was designed. This procedure generates independent monthly samples of the population of interest. The advantages and constraints involved in the methodology are discussed.

INTRODUCTION

Existing surveillance activities of the Human Immunodeficiency Virus (HIV) epidemic have focused mainly on at-risk populations which are in contact with health organizations such as addicts entering drug treatment units, clients attending Sexually Transmitted Disease (STD) clinics, or hospital admissions. Populations which are not likely to utilize health services or other institutional settings on a regular basis are "hidden" from most epidemiological data collection systems. This is especially true of drug addicts. It is known that only a small proportion of drug addicts use drug treatment services and several studies have shown that injection drug users (IDUs) not in treatment report more frequent risk behaviors and higher HIV seropositivity rates than those studied while attending treatment programs (Franceschi et al., 1988; McCusker, Koblin, Lewis & Sullivan, 1990). These facts have prompted the resurgence of community outreach techniques combining epidemiological as well as intervention objectives.

The Cooperative Agreement Program for research in AIDS Community-Based Outreach and Intervention of the National Institute on Drug Abuse (NIDA) has been established with two interrelated objectives: (a) to establish a system for monitoring trends in the nature and extent of HIV-related risk-taking behaviors and in levels of HIV seropositivity in out-of-treatment crack and injection drug users, and (b) to assess the efficacy of interventions in reducing risk behaviors in these populations. Monitoring behaviors and serostatus in street addicts requires the recruitment and assessment of successive samples of the population. Sampling street addicts presents a number of difficult methodological problems. Random sampling is most often not feasible. To date, most studies have utilized various types of convenience samples. While rich in content and inexpensive to implement, convenience samples are vulnerable to a variety of selection biases.

Targeted sampling has proven effective in reaching systematically selected samples of injection drug users. Targeted sampling is defined as "a purposeful, systematic method by which controlled lists of specific populations (i.e., zip codes, census tracks, census blocks) are developed and detailed plans are designed to recruit an adequate number of cases within each of the targets." Watters and Biernacki (1989) recognize that this is not a strictly random sample but it is far more rigorous than the more widespread convenience sampling. Its principal advantage is the careful delineation of methods by which respondents are identified and selected for interview. The target populations are also well defined.

The weakness in the targeted sampling strategy is that the linkage between the target population and the population actually sampled is not readily amenable to mathematical analysis. The strength of random sampling is that the linkages become known probabilities which can be analyzed. Moreover, the assumptions associated with probability samples are readily operationalized in terms of response rates, sampling rates, coverage errors, and selection bias. These qualities, in conjunction with sampling errors, have been the reason investigators undertake these logistically rigorous projects. This paper is an effort to describe the strategies used to implement this method of sampling among crack and injection drug users in San Juan, Puerto Rico. Particular emphasis is made on the compromises that were required. These compromises reflect not only the practical issues of detecting, recruiting, and interviewing injection drug users, but also the dangers inherent in this type of investigation.

SAMPLING CONSTRAINTS

The sampling plan designed for the San Juan site establishes subject recruitment procedures that allow generalization to larger population groups, and measurement of trends in risk behaviors and HIV seropositivity. The proposed procedures aim to reduce selection bias to the greatest extent possible, given the resources and limitations present. The sample selection outlined in this plan also attempts to broaden access to populations under study as much as feasible.

Realistically, we needed to limit the nature of our target population in three areas. First and most importantly, we restricted our attention to pedestrian drug purchasers. We know that perhaps as many as 40% of drug users make purchases without leaving their automobile. Our previous experience in the field has demonstrated that these individuals are nearly impossible to contact. A second limitation regards drug purchases made in late evening or early morning hours. The environment after dark is quite violent. We did not feel an appropriate level of security could be maintained for recruiters. Based on subjective field experience, we believe that after dark purchases are made primarily by individuals who also make daylight purchases, so only those individuals who are exclusively nocturnal have been excluded from our frame. Finally, we assumed that areas of drug purchases remain stable sources for users for periods of at least one month.

Based on these considerations, we developed a three-stage sampling strategy. The first was the relatively simple random sampling of daylight time periods each month. One hour periods were believed adequate periods. The second stage was the selection of recruitment sites. The third and final stage was the selection of crack and injection drug users for recruitment.

COPPING AREAS AS SAMPLING AND RECRUITMENT SITES

Outreachers of the Puerto Rico Cooperative Agreement Project identified specific points within communities where drugs are sold, where there are special car services, crack houses, shooting galleries, and where needles and other drug equipment can be purchased. These complex drug service territories are termed *copping areas* and are the focus of our targeted area sample. Information has been also collected regarding the location, size, structure, and complexity of copping areas (see Map of Copping Areas and Tables 1 and 2).

From a community perspective, our previous research experience suggests that the street copping areas in San Juan offer certain clear advantages as sampling and recruitment sites. Drug-related activities at copping areas are easily identifiable and can be observed. Copping areas provide drug users a social context in which they can interact and engage in drug-buying and drug-using routines. Thus,

Table 1

Observed Location, Size, Gang Affiliation, and Hours of Operation of Drug Copping Areas In Six Municipalities of the San Juan Metropolitan Area (N = 64)

OCTOBER 1991 - FEBRUARY 1992

Characteristics	N	%
Municipality of Location		
San Juan	33	51.6
Carolina	13	20.3
Trujillo Alto	3	4.7
Guaynabo	5	7.8
Bayamón	7	10.9
Cataño	3	4.7
Type of Neighborhood		
Public Housing Project	52	81.3
Other Urban Neighborhood	12	18.7
Size (Number of Street Dealers)[a]		
1 - 3	20	31.7
4 - 6	23	36.5
≥ 7	20	31.7
Gang Affiliation		
Ñetas	57	89.1
Insectos	7	10.9
Hours of Operation		
24 Hours	39	60.9
Daylight Hours	25	39.1

[a] Information missing in one case.

Table 2

Observed Drugs and Related Services Available at Drug Copping Areas in Six Municipalities of the San Juan Metropolitan Area (N = 64)

OCTOBER 1991 - FEBRUARY 1992

Characteristics	N	%
Types of Drugs Sold[a]		
Heroin	35	54.7
Cocaine	55	85.9
Crack	44	68.8
Marihuana	51	79.7
Other	13	20.3
Related Services[a]		
Car Service	50	78.1
Shooting Gallery	33	51.6
Crack Pipes for Sale	8	12.5
Crack Houses	14	21.9
Needles/Syringes for Sale	23	35.9

[a] Numbers do not add up, copping areas might sell more than one type of drug

and offer more than one related service.

copping areas constitute a setting where drug users can be identified and approached.

To identify and characterize the copping areas within the San Juan metropolitan area, we used the following sources of information:

MAP OF COPPING AREAS

CONTINUOUS CARE FOR THE PREVENTION OF HIV RISK BEHAVIORS

TARGETED AREA AND LOCATION OF COPPING AREAS

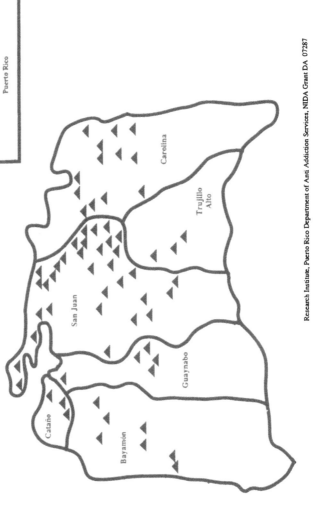

Research Institute, Puerto Rico Department of Anti Addiction Services, NIDA Grant DA 07287

- Acquired Immune Deficiency Syndrome (AIDS) registry by municipality
- Sexually Transmitted Disease (STD) registry by municipality
- Management Information System (MIS) data on drug injectors and crack users entering the drug treatment system of DAAS
- Police records of the San Juan Metropolitan Area
- Census data (to estimate per capita rates of AIDS and Syphilis cases, and treatment admissions of crack and Intravenous Drug Users [IDUs])
- Visual inspection of copping areas

The Puerto Rico AIDS registry, the treatment system dataset, and the STD registry have helped in selecting the minor civil divisions (MCDs) within the San Juan Metropolitan Area most likely to have the highest prevalence of copping areas (see Puerto Rico Maps 1 through 4). We corroborated these data with data from the Puerto Rico AIDS Prevention Project (PRAPP; data from this project is included in the National AIDS Demonstration Research Program (NADR) of NIDA). However, PRAPP was more useful in helping identify specific sites, within the communities or neighborhoods of MCDs, with high prevalence of HIV infection. Moreover, recruiter observation in a copping area allowed us to reliably estimate the number of users as well as gender and age distribution.

As a geographical unit, MCDs cover wide areas and do not provide the detailed neighborhood and demographic information needed to characterize the components of the targeted population. In addition, information broken down by location of residence may not correspond to the recruitment location. While the San Juan Metropolitan Area covers a small geographical area (775 sq. miles), it is very densely inhabited (2,179.5 persons per sq. mile). Daily mobility within the metropolitan area by public or private transportation is facilitated by small distances, a high degree of urbanization, and the relative non-existence of ethnic or racial geographical boundaries. Thus, street addicts in San Juan move from one neighborhood to another while pursuing a daily routine of drug buying and using. Although the NADR San Juan data shows some important differences among injection drug users recruited in different parts of the city, we have also found that substantial numbers of

MAP 1

SYPHILIS CASES REGISTERED IN 1990-91 AS RATES
PER CAPITA OF MUNICIPALITY OF RESIDENCE

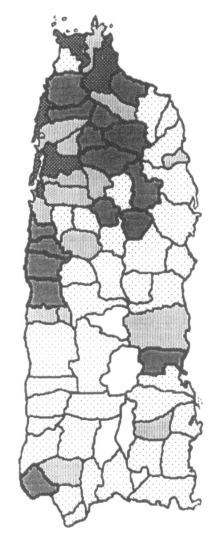

LEGEND: PER CAPITA RATES (PER 100,000 POPULATION)

☐ < 30 CASES   91-120 CASES

☐ 31-60 CASES   ≥ 121 CASES

☐ 61-90 CASES   ☐ NO CASES REGISTERED

N = 1,879 CASES

Source: STD Control Program, P. R. Health Department, 1991

MAP 2

INJECTION DRUG USERS ADMITTED TO DRUG TREATMENT IN 1990-1991
AS RATES PER CAPITA OF MUNICIPALITY OR RESIDENCE

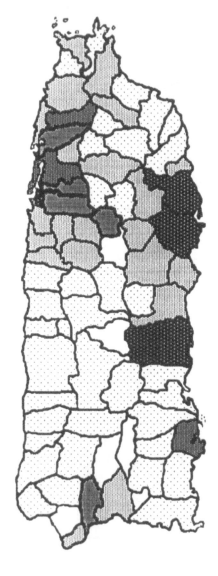

LEGEND: PER CAPITA RATES (PER 100,000 POPULATION)

☐ ≤ 30 CASES   ■ 91-120 CASES
▒ 31-60 CASES   ▓ ≥ 121 CASES
▓ 61-90 CASES   ☐ NO CASES ADMITTED

N = 1,978 CASES

Source: Puerto Rico Department of Anti Addiction Services, 1991

MAP 3

CRACK USERS ADMITTED TO DRUG TREATMENT IN 1990-91 AS RATES
PER CAPITA OF MUNICIPALITY OF RESIDENCE

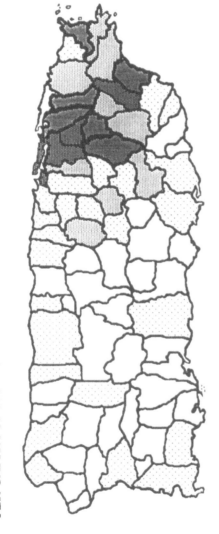

LEGEND: PER CAPITA RATES (PER 100,000 POPULATION)

☐ < 10 CASES
▨ 10-19 CASES
▨ 20-29 CASES

■ ≥ 30 CASES
☐ NO CASES ADMITTED

N = 449 ADMISSIONS

Source: Puerto Rico Department of Anti Addiction Services, 1991

MAP 4

AIDS CASES ATTRIBUTED TO INJECTION DRUG USE REPORTED IN 1990 AS RATES PER CAPITA OF MUNICIPALITY

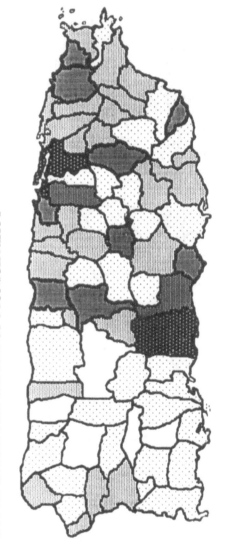

LEGEND: PER CAPITA RATES (PER 100,000 POPULATION)

- 1-15 CASES
- 16-30 CASES
- 31-45 CASES
- 46-60 CASES
- 61-75 CASES
- NO CASES REGISTERED

N = 1,133 CASES

Source: Central Office for AIDS Issues, P. R. Health Department, 1991

participants recruited in one area were not residents of the same area. Therefore, a convenience sample with quotas for gender, age, or type of drug used (crack vs. injected), which reflects municipality of residence may be biased when compared to the groups found in copping areas.

Sampling Procedures

The copping areas in San Juan will be utilized as first stage clustering sampling units. This requires preparing a complete list of all operating areas (see STEP 1 following). Subjects will be recruited from samples of copping areas.

The proposed sampling method will generate independent monthly samples of the populations under study. The samples are a three-stage probability sample of crack and injection drug users buying and/or using drugs at copping areas in the San Juan Metropolitan Area. Each month a fixed number of copping areas and recruitment days and times are selected at random. On the designated day and time outreach workers visit selected copping areas and estimate the number of buyers in the area. A buyer is then selected at random using standard Kish selection tables. The selected individual is invited to participate and a written appointment will be handed to him. Outreach workers follow-up and encourage participation from the selected users for up to thirty days. Selected individuals who refuse to participate or who do not complete the assessment interview will be considered non-respondents.

Sampling procedures will require the following steps to be executed on a monthly basis:

STEP 1. Identify Copping Areas (M)

During October 1991 to February 1992, the outreach staff identified and characterized the copping areas of the San Juan Metro Area (see Map of Copping Areas and Tables 1 and 2). Wholesale distribution operations and areas where Marihuana was the only drug for sale were defined as ineligible and not included in the sample frame. To date 64 areas have been identified and documented. Observable indicators, such as number of drug dealers, drugs for sale, and available drug use-related services, have been recorded. The listing of copping areas has been verified with a list furnished by the Police Department. This verified list comprises the sampling frame of copping areas from which a fixed number will be randomly selected on a monthly basis. The list is to be updated monthly as outreachers report on new areas not previously identified, or old ones closed down. The monthly listing of operating areas should constitute the most complete and exhaustive list of copping areas available.

STEP 2. *Randomly Select m Number of Copping Areas and t Recruitment Days and Times Each Month*

The number of areas selected will depend mainly on the available resources. It is expected that one outreach staff will be able to select and recruit the monthly sample in one area. Based on this assumption we are currently planning on a sample size of 6 copping areas a month. Recruitment at each copping area will occur at randomly selected days and times. Ten entry moments (t) will be selected for each copping area based on the daylight hours of operation previously observed for each area (T).

STEP 3. *"Count" Area Users (N) on Randomly Selected Day and Time*

Once in the designated area, outreachers will estimate, through observation, the number of users buying and using drugs. This estimate will be used to calculate the selection probability of the sampled subjects. The reliability of these estimates is currently being studied. For estimation purposes crack and injection drug users recruited at a copping area on a given month will be weighted by the inverse probability of selection. An alternative approach to estimating the number of users in an area could be the use of the number of dealers as an indicator of the size of the drug purchasing population. Analyses of the strength of association between counts of users and counts of dealers are also being examined.

STEP 4. *Select 1 User at Random from Each Selected Copping Area (m) and Day and Time (t)*

Project participants will be selected at random from the total individuals observed at each entry point. Kish type tables will be used to select individuals. Selected individuals who cannot be approached, who refuse to participate, or who fail to complete the assessment interview will be considered non-respondents. Ten entry moments for 6 areas will result in a recruitment quota of 60 participants a month. An additional advantage of this methodology is the possibility of knowing non-response rates.

Estimation Procedures

The sampling methodology outlined above will result in monthly estimates of the risk behaviors of interest and HIV serostatus. Standard deviations and standard errors can also be estimated utilizing available statistical software for complex samples such as PC-CARP or SAS SUDAN. Given the small sample sizes, monthly estimates could be rather unstable. Nevertheless, monthly estimates can be combined into 3, 6, or 12 month periods to increase precision.

REFERENCES

Franceschi, S., Tirelli, U., Vaccher, E., Serraino, D., Crovatto, M., De Paoli, P., Diodato, S., La Vecchia, C., Decarli, A., & Monfardini, S. (1988). Risk factors for HIV infection in drug addicts from the northeast of Italy. *International Journal of Epidemiology, 17,* 162-167.

McCusker, J., Koblin, B., Lewis, B.F., & Sullivan, J. (1990). Demographic characteristics, risk behaviors, and HIV seroprevalence among intravenous drug users by site of contact: Results from a community-wide HIV surveillance project. *American Journal of Public Health, 80,* 1062-7.

Watters, J.K., & Biernacki, P. (1989). Targeted sampling: Options for the study of hidden populations. *Social Problems, 36,* 416-430.

Drug Use and HIV Risk
in Alaska Natives

Dennis G. Fisher, PhD
Henry H. Cagle, BS
Patricia J. Wilson, MSN

Little has been published about Alaska Natives or American Indians and their risk for Human Immunodeficiency Virus (HIV) (Estrada, Erickson, Stevens, & Fernandez, 1990; Rowell, 1990). Some small exploratory studies of HIV seroprevalence among Alaska Natives have been done (Davidson, Kaplan, Hartley, Lairmore, & Lanier, 1990; Robert-Guroff et al., 1985), but no published behavioral studies. There has been a report that intravenous cocaine and amphetamine use was the major route of transmission in an

Dennis G. Fisher is Director of the Center for Alcohol and Addiction Studies at University of Alaska Anchorage. Henry H. Cagle and Patricia J. Wilson are also affiliated with the Center for Alcohol and Addiction Studies.

Appreciation for assistance with this project is gratefully given to Mark Johnson, Alice Baer, Sherry Donnelly, Dawn Davis, Ken Brooks, Mont Hadley and Grace Reynolds.

This research was supported in part by grant number 1 U01 DA07290 from the National Institute on Drug Abuse.

Requests for reprints should be sent to Dennis G. Fisher, Center for Alcohol and Addiction Studies, University of Alaska Anchorage, 3211 Providence Drive, Anchorage, AK 99508.

[Haworth co-indexing entry note]: "Drug Use and HIV Risk in Alaska Natives." Fisher, Dennis G., Henry H. Cagle, and Patricia J. Wilson. Co-published simultaneously in *Drugs & Society* (The Haworth Press, Inc.) Vol. 7, No. 3/4, 1993, pp. 107-117; and: *AIDS and Community-Based Drug Intervention Programs: Evaluation and Outreach* (ed: Dennis G. Fisher, and Richard Needle) The Haworth Press, Inc., 1993, pp. 107-117. Multiple copies of this article/chapter may be purchased from The Haworth Document Delivery Center [1-800-3-HAWORTH; 9:00 a.m. - 5:00 p.m. (EST)].

Copyright © 1993 by Taylor & Francis

epidemic of hepatitis B among American Indians (Harding, Helgerson, & Damrow, 1992). The first paper published on intravenous drug use (IVDU) in Alaska concluded that Alaska has a major problem with IVDU and that this could be an important vector of HIV transmission into the non-IVDU population of the state (Fisher, Wilson, & Brause, 1990). A recent master's thesis (Tarrant, 1992) found that Blacks, Natives, and Hispanics were overrepresented in a sample of community health outreach worker contacts of IVDUs and their sex partners. Also reported was the finding that Alaska Native IVDUs were younger than other ethnic groups. Tarrant suggested this indicates that drug use is a recent phenomenon in the Native community.

Conway, Hooper, and St. Louis (1989) found that HIV seroprevalence is higher for Native Americans than the cumulative incidence of AIDS in this group. They suggest that there is either: widespread racial misclassification, or more recent entrance of HIV into this population.

The concern about IVDU among the American Indian/Alaska Native (AI/AN) group derives from the high levels of drug use among this group, and the frequency of their high risk behaviors (Conway et al., 1992; Estrada et al., 1990; Fisher & Booker, 1990; Rowell, 1990). These concerns may be validated by reports that the increase in diagnosed AIDS cases from 1989 to 1990 was higher among the AI/AN group than any other ethnic group (Melter, Conway, & Stehr-Green, 1991).

FEMALE SPECIFICS

In general, women are the fastest growing group of people with AIDS (Shayne & Kaplan, 1991). In particular, those who are poor and are ethnic minorities have been afflicted. There are two predominant routes by which women in America are becoming infected with HIV. The first is through IVDU, and the second is by having unprotected sex with an infected male IVDU (Cohen, Hauer, & Wofsy, 1989; Des Jarlais, Chamberland, Yancovitz, Weinberg, & Friedman, 1984). Klee, Faugier, Hayes, Boulton, and Morris (1990) found that injection drug users who share their injection equipment are less likely to use condoms than non-sharing injectors. The female sex partners of injection drug users have been the subject of some attention and increased risk has been observed for Black female sex partners of injection drug users (Corby, Wolitski, Thornton-Johnson, & Tanner, 1991). The risk behaviors of AI/AN women have not been as well investigated as those for Black women.

Melter and Stehr-Green (1990) report that the distribution of Acquired Immune Deficiency Syndrome (AIDS) cases for the AI/AN group is unique in that it is the only ethnic group that has more female than male IVDUs. Other ethnic groups have consistently reported more male than female drug users in a variety of studies, but Beauvais, Oetting, Wolf, and Edwards (1989) appear to corroborate the notion of equal sex ratios of drug users among AI/AN in that their data show that female subjects use drugs at the same rate as the male subjects.

METHOD

Subjects

Subjects were recruited within the Municipality of Anchorage Alaska using a targeted sampling strategy (Watters & Biernacki, 1989). The data collection took place from October 1991 through April 1992, at the Drug Abuse Research Field Station (DARFS) in Anchorage, Alaska. In order to be eligible for the study a subject had to: (a) be eighteen years of age or older, (b) test positive for either cocaine, morphine, or amphetamine on a urine test (Roche Diagnostics), and/or (c) present visible "track" marks indicative of recent injection drug use, and (d) not have been in drug or alcohol treatment within the last 30 days.

Instruments

The major data collection instrument was the Risk Behavior Assessment (RBA). This instrument focuses on high risk behaviors for HIV. It has been subject to extensive reliability testing (Needle et al., 1992). A supplemental questionnaire was also used. This supplemental questionnaire asked about dates of first injection, locations of first and last injection (city and state), and drug of choice.

RESULTS

There are 352 interviewees of whom 62 (17.33%) are self-identified Alaska Natives. Figure 1 shows the ethnic distribution of our sample (labeled DARFS) in comparison with the overall ethnic distribution of the Municipality of Anchorage (Fison et al., 1991). Whites and Asians are underrepresented in our sample, whereas Blacks and Natives are overrepresented. Over 95% of all interviewees reported that their sexual preference is heterosexual. The Alaska Natives (M = 30.67 years) are significantly younger than the non-natives (M = 34.97 years) $t(93.2)$ = 4.64, p = .0001. There is a greater proportion of female interviewees among the Alaska Natives than there is for the other two ethnic groups $X^2(1, N = 352)$ = 12.746, p = .000. There are almost equal numbers of female and male Alaska Natives in the sample. The Alaska Natives reported having significantly lower income than the non-natives $t(87.7)$ = 1.99, p = .049. As measured on an ordinal scale of 8th grade, less than high school, GED, high school graduate, trade school, some college, and college graduate, the Alaska Natives are significantly lower than the other two ethnicities (Kruskal-Wallis approximation) $X^2(2)$ = 25.718, p = .0001.

When asked the question "Has a doctor or a nurse ever told you that you have had hepatitis B?" the Alaska Natives are significantly more likely to report in the affirmative than non-natives $X^2(1, N = 351)$ = 6.889, p = . 009.

When route of administration (intravenous, or smoking) is examined by ethnicity, it is apparent that Blacks are significantly more likely to be smokers, whereas Whites and Natives are about equally split between smoking and injection drug use $X^2(2, N = 350)$ = 75.833, p = .000. Of the 62 Alaska Natives in the sample, 39 report that they have never injected drugs. When asked "Where were you when you first shot drugs?" 29 of the Alaska Natives report that they were in Alaska, 3 in California, 2 in Washington state, and one each in New Mexico, Ohio, Oregon, Japan, and VietNam. Of those who reported that they were in Alaska, 25 said that they were in

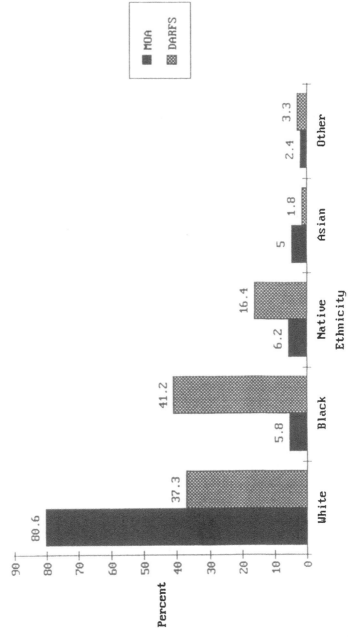

FIGURE 1. Ethnic Distribution of Municipality of Anchorage (MOA) as Compared with Drug Abuse Research Field Station (DARFS) through September 30, 1992. N = 451

Anchorage, and one each in Fairbanks, Kodiak, McGrath, and Petersberg. When asked "Where were you when you last shot drugs?" 34 of the Alaska Natives report that they were in Alaska, and one each in California, Oregon, and Washington state. When asked where they were right before they came to Alaska, five report California, two Hawaii, and one each in Arizona, Kansas, New York, Oklahoma, and Washington state. Twenty-nine of the Alaska Natives report that their drug of choice is cocaine, three report heroin, two other opiates, and three other drugs.

There are more Alaska Native injectors who are female than male. Both Blacks and Whites have several times more male as compared to female injectors $X^2(2, N = 108) = 9.463, p = .009$. The reversal of this gender relationship is noteworthy.

The mean number of sex partners in the last 30 days is lower for the Alaska Natives than it is for the non-natives, but not significantly so. The number of sex partners in the last 30 days who were drug injectors is significantly higher for the Alaska Natives ($M = 0.79$) as compared to the non-natives ($M = 0.38$) $t(59.6) = 2.07, p = .0428$. The reason why these means are less than unity is because they include respondents who did not have sex with drug injectors. When the number of sex partners in the last 30 days who were drug injectors is used as the numerator, and the total number of sex partners in the last 30 days is used as the denominator, the quotient is the percent of sex partners in the last 30 days who were drug injectors. This value, percent of sex partners who were injectors, was used as a dependent variable in a two-way full factorial ANOVA. We used PROC GLM type III sums of square because of unequal cell sizes (SAS Institute Inc. [SAS], 1988). Interviewees who reported abstinence in the last 30 days were deleted from the analysis. There is a main effect of ethnicity $F(2, 259) = 12.60, p = .001$, but neither is there a main effect of sex, nor an ethnicity by sex interaction. Referring to Figure 2 it is clear that the Blacks are significantly lower than the other two ethnicities. It is also noteworthy that, by far, the group with the highest percentage is the female Alaska Natives.

Examining just the female Alaska Native interviewees, a comparison of injectors with smokers shows that, as expected, the injectors ($M = 57.9\%$) have a higher percentage of injecting sex partners

FIGURE 2. Percent of Sex Partners in the Last 30 Days Who Were Injectors. N = 388

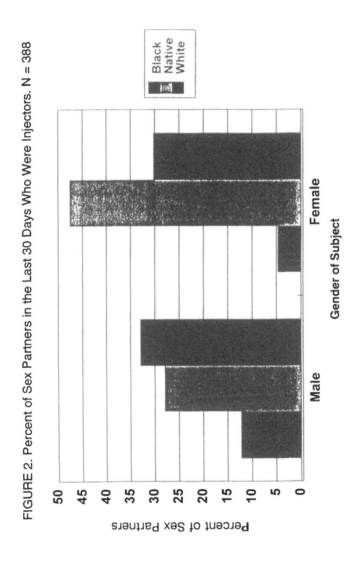

than the smokers (M = 39.3%), of particular interest is that the female Alaska Native smokers have a higher mean percentage than any other sex-ethnic group. The sex, that is, vaginal, oral and anal, that the female Alaska Natives are having is predominantly unprotected sex. Condom use is reported at the following rates: vaginal 12%, oral 5%, and anal 25%. In the 30 days prior to interview, vaginal sex is the most frequent type of sexual activity (M = 15.33, SD = 13.82).

DISCUSSION

The Alaska Natives in our sample are younger than the non-natives. This corroborates a finding by Tarrant (1992). It may be that Natives have only recently begun moving to both smoking and injecting cocaine, as their historical drug of abuse has been alcohol. We may see a younger age of HIV infection associated with drug use in this population if HIV has only recently entered the AI/AN population as Conway et al. (1989) have suggested.

The finding concerning hepatitis B is not surprising as this disease has been at high levels in this population for decades (Arctic Investigations Laboratory [AIL], 1986; Tower, 1987). Of particular concern, is the potential for a hepatitis B epidemic in non-native needle users who share needles with Alaska Native needle users who are infectious for hepatitis B.

The geographical data on the Alaska Native needle users are important because they document the West Coast influence on the drug use in Alaska. If only states that have at least two mentions are listed, then the states are: California, Oregon, Washington, and Hawaii. This is very consistent with anecdotal information concerning drug terminology and drug using practices. Alaska drug use is heavily influenced by conditions along the Pacific Coast and Hawaii.

Another important point is that some Alaska Natives reported they first injected drugs in Alaskan locations outside of Anchorage. This finding means the belief that intravenous drug use takes place only in Anchorage and not in other Alaskan cities is incorrect: It takes place in smaller cities, villages, and fishing and logging communities as well.

The finding that there are more Alaska Native female injectors than Alaska Native male injectors is consistent with the general findings of others (Beauvais et al., 1989; Metler & Stehr-Green, 1990). This is one major way that Alaska Native women are at risk for HIV infection, the extent of which has not been given adequate attention in the literature. Drug use in general, and injection drug use in particular, may be a recent phenomenon for Alaska Natives. Nonetheless, the high proportion of needle users among female Alaska Native subjects is an important point that should not be ignored in designing culturally-appropriate HIV/AIDS prevention materials and interventions.

The finding that female Alaska Natives have a greater percentage of their sex partners who are needle users than any other sex-race group in our sample is also a finding that is disturbing. This is true even for those women who are not themselves needle users. A large percentage of the sexual contacts did not involve the use of condoms or other latex barrier protective methods.

The Alaska Native women in our sample are at especially high risk of HIV infection through injection drug use, and having unprotected sex with injection drug users. These behaviors need to be given more attention in the educational materials and processes provided to these individuals. Not only is more investigation into the sexual and drug using behaviors of female Alaska Natives called for, but also the social networks of these women and their sexual and injection partners need to be delineated.

REFERENCES

Arctic Investigations Laboratory. (1986, March 31). *Arctic investigations laboratory: Description of programs 1984/1986.* Anchorage, AK: Center for Infectious Diseases, Centers for Disease Control.

Beauvais, F., Oetting, E. R., Wolf, W., & Edwards, R. W. (1989, May). American Indian youth and drugs, 1976-87: A continuing problem. *American Journal of Public Health, 79*(5), 634-636.

Cohen, J. B., Hauer, L. B., & Wofsy, C. B. (1989). Women and IV drugs: Parenteral and heterosexual transmission of Human Immunodeficiency Virus. *The Journal of Drug Issues, 19*(1), 39-56.

Conway, G. A., Ambrose, T. J., Epstein, M. R., Chase, E., Johannes, P., Hooper, E. Y., & Helgerson, S. D. (1992, May). Prevalence of HIV and AIDS in American Indians and Alaska Natives. *The IHS Primary Care Provider, 17*(5), 65-70.

Conway, G. A., Hooper, E. Y., & St. Louis, M. E. (1989, June 4-9). Risk of AIDS and HIV infection in American Indians and Alaska Natives. *International AIDS Conference*, *5*, 123. (abstract no. W.A.P.23)

Corby, N. H., Wolitski, R. J., Thornton-Johnson, S., & Tanner, W. M. (1991, Winter). AIDS knowledge, perception of risk, and behaviors among female sex partners of injection drug users. *AIDS Education and Prevention*, *3*(4), 353-366.

Davidson, M., Kaplan, J. E., Hartley, T. M., Lairmore, M. D., & Lanier, A. P. (1990, February). Prevalence of HTLV-I in Alaska Natives [Letter to the editor]. *The Journal of Infectious Diseases*, *161*(2), 359-360.

Des Jarlais, D. C., Chamberland, M. E., Yancovitz, S. R., Weinberg, P., & Friedman, S. R. (1984, December 8). Heterosexual partners: A large risk group for AIDS [Letter to the editor]. *The Lancet*, *2*(8415), 1346-1347.

Estrada, A. L., Erickson, J. R., Stevens, S., & Fernandez, M. (1990, June 22). HIV risk behaviors among native American IVDU's. *International AIDS Conference*, *2*, 270. (F.C.757)

Fisher, D. G., & Booker, J. M. (1990). Drug abuse in Alaska: Myths versus reality. *Psychology of Addictive Behaviors*, *4*(1), 2-5.

Fisher, D. G., Wilson, P. J., & Brause, J. (1990). Intravenous drug use in Alaska. *Drugs & Society*, *5*(1/2), 9-20.

Fison, S. R., Collins, M. P., Yang, X., Ameen, L. K., Hunt, D., & Whitelaw, D. (Eds.). (1991, June). *Anchorage indicators: A socioeconomic review*. Anchorage, AK: Municipality of Anchorage. (Department of Economic Development and Planning)

Harding, R., Helgerson, S. D., & Damrow, T. (1992, January 10). Hepatitis B and injecting-drug use among American Indians: Montana, 1989-1990. *Morbidity and Mortality Weekly Report*, *41*(1), 13-14.

Klee, H., Faugier, J., Hayes, C., Boulton, T., & Morris, J. (1990). Sexual partners of injecting drug users: The risk of HIV infection. *British Journal of Addictions*, *85*, 413-418.

Metler, R., Conway, G. A., & Stehr-Green, J. (1991). AIDS surveillance among American Indians and Alaska Natives. *American Journal of Public Health*, *81*(11), 1469-1471.

Meter, R., & Stehr-Green, J. (1990, June 20-23). AIDS surveillance among American Indians and Alaskan Natives. *International AIDS Conference*, *6*(1), 300. (Th.C.701)

Needle, R., Weatherby, N., Brown, B. S., Booth, R., Williams, M. L., Watters, J., Andersen, M., Chitwood, D. D., Fisher, D. G., Cesari, H., & Braunstein, M. (1992). *The reliability of self-reported HIV risk behaviors of injection and non-injection drug users.*

Robert-Guroff, M., Clark, J., Lanier, A. P., Beckman, G., Melbye, M., Ebbesen, P., Blattner, W. A., & Gallo, R. C. (1985). Prevalence of HTLV-I in Arctic Regions. *International Journal of Cancer*, *36*, 651-655.

Rowell, R. M. (1990). Warning signs: Intravenous drug abuse among American Indians/Alaskan Natives. *Drugs & Society*, *5*(1/2), 21-35.

SAS Institute Inc. (1988). *SAS/STAT User's Guide* (release 6.03 edition). Cary, NC: SAS Institute.

Shayne, V. T., & Kaplan, B. J. (1991). Double victims: Poor women and AIDS. *Women's Health, 17*(1), 21-37.

Tarrant, D. L. (1992). *A description of intravenous drug users not in treatment and their sex partners in Anchorage, Alaska.* Unpublished master's thesis, University of Alaska Anchorage. Anchorage.

Tower, E. A. (1987). Alaska state hepatitis B program: Past, present and future. *Alaska Medicine, 29*(1), 1-8.

Watters, J. K., & Biernacki, P. (1989). Targeted sampling: Options for the study of hidden populations. *Social Problems, 36*(4), 416-430.

Behavior Change Strategies
for Women at High Risk for HIV

Sherry Deren, PhD
Mark Beardsley, RhD
Stephanie Tortu, PhD
Rees Davis, PhD
Michael Clatts, PhD

As of December 1991, East Harlem in New York City accounted for 1,186 cases of Acquired Immunodeficiency Syndrome (AIDS) among adults. The majority of these cases, 62% of the cases among men and 69% of the cases among women, were related to the individual being an injection drug user. An additional 23% of the female cases were among women who were the sex partner of an intravenous drug user (N.Y.C., 1992). The N.Y.C. Health Services Administration, in 1990, estimated the percent of the adult population in New York City, by neighborhood, that was Human Immunodeficiency Virus (HIV) infected. This report estimated the highest rate in New York City to be in East Harlem, with a rate of 13.4-17.9%

Sherry Deren, Mark Beardsley, Stephanie Tortu, Rees Davis, and Michael Clatts are affiliated with the National Development and Research Institutes, Inc., New York, NY.

This article is based on a paper presented at the AIDS Prevention Symposium, University of Alaska, Anchorage, May 1992.

[Haworth co-indexing entry note]: "Behavior Change Strategies for Women at High Risk for HIV." Deren, Sherry et al. Co-published simultaneously in *Drugs & Society* (The Haworth Press, Inc.) Vol. 7, No. 3/4, 1993, pp. 119-128; and: *AIDS and Community-Based Intervention Drug Programs: Evaluation and Outreach* (ed: Dennis G. Fisher, and Richard Needle) The Haworth Press, Inc., 1993, pp. 119-128. Multiple copies of this article/chapter may be purchased from The Haworth Document Delivery Center [1-800-3-HAWORTH; 9:00 a.m. - 5:00 p.m. (EST)].

Copyright © 1993 by Taylor & Francis

of the adult population being HIV infected (HSA/NYC, 1990). The impact of this magnitude of HIV infection, and the potential for its transmission throughout the community, calls for increased and extensive HIV prevention efforts, particularly among those most at risk. Three goals of these efforts, all goals of the East Harlem project to be discussed in this paper, are as follows: (a) to prevent high risk individuals from getting infected; (b) if already infected, to teach behaviors which will prevent them from transmitting the virus; and c) if already infected, to learn specific health-related skills which may help retard the progression from HIV infection to an AIDS diagnosis.

It is particularly important to develop behavior change strategies for high-risk women in East Harlem. As of December 1991, women represented approximately 10% of the AIDS cases in the United States (Center for Disease Control [CDC], 1992); in East Harlem women represent almost one-quarter (23%) of the total AIDS cases among adults (N.Y.C., 1991). Prevention efforts targeted to women can impact on HIV rates among women and on the increasing number of pediatric AIDS cases due to vertical transmission of HIV to newborns.

The Harlem AIDS Project (HAP) was funded by the National Institute on Drug Abuse as one of the National AIDS Demonstration and Research (NADR) projects, which were located in over 60 locations throughout the United States.

HAP focused on injection drug users and sex partners of injection drug users throughout Harlem and recruited clients to participate in research interviews and an AIDS prevention effort from 1989 through 1991 (for a detailed description of the methods of this intervention see Deren, 1989). The current cooperative agreement project focuses specifically on East Harlem. This paper will briefly summarize: (a) the original HAP intervention; (b) some of the data about the women who participated in HAP; and (c) a revised intervention, based on the HAP findings.

METHOD

HAP Intervention

As with all NADR projects, both standard and enhanced interventions were developed. Clients participated in a baseline interview and were then assigned to an intervention. Clients in the standard intervention participated in one AIDS Education Group, focussing on AIDS transmission and risk reduction. At the end of the first session clients were informed about the availability of a referral service and individual counseling related to risk reduction. Clients randomly assigned to the Enhanced intervention participated in two additional sessions, based on a cognitive-behavioral social learning model, which involved demonstrating skills necessary for risk reduction and giving clients the opportunity to practice these skills in the group (see Table 1).

The components of the social learning model (demonstration, observation, practice and reinforcement; Bandura, 1977) are ideally suited for a group context and increase self efficacy, a critical factor in successful AIDS prevention efforts (Bandura, 1987). Hartgers, Van den Hoek, Coutinho, and Van Der Pligt (1990) recommended that prevention efforts focus on enhancing self-efficacy. Furthermore, providing information-only approaches without skill devel-

Table 1. HAP Intervention

Session 1: GOAL: AIDS Overview (For Standard and Enhanced)

> Basic Information: AIDS Transmission and Prevention
> Self assessment of risk
> AIDS is preventable
> Introduction of referral coordinator

Sessions 2 and 3: GOAL: Skill Development (Enhanced Only)

> Session 2:
> Learn behaviors which can reduce risk
> Discuss alternative behaviors
> Demonstration and practice: needle cleaning and condom use

> Session 3:
> Learn to use risk reduction behaviors
> Discuss methods of using these behaviors
> Practice negotiation techniques

opment, has not been greatly successful in modifying risk behaviors. Skills taught in the HAP enhanced intervention were needle cleaning, condom use, and the negotiation techniques needed to practice risk reduction.

Characteristics of Women Participating in HAP

A total of 653 women participated in HAP, and selected demographic characteristics are presented in Table 2. The women were primarily minority (Afro-American and Hispanic), about two-thirds were injection drug users (IDUs) and one-third were sexual partners of injection drug users (SPs). The poor social and economic circumstances experienced by these women are indicated by some of the

Table 2. Demographic Characteristics of HAP Women (N=624)*

Ethnicity:	African-American: 71%	Hispanic : 25%
Mean Age:	33	
Target Populaton:	IDUs: 65%	Sexual Partners: 35%
Jail experience:	54%	
HS graduate:	45%	
Employment:	79% unemployed	
Current income sources:	Welfare- 59% Spouse/sex partner-30% Illegal activities - 38%	

*The total N for women was 653; the demographic information presented is based only on Afro-american and Hispanic women, a total N of 624.

demographic and economic characteristics summarized in Table 2. For example, over half (54%) had previously been in jail, less than half were high school graduates (45%) and the majority were unemployed (79%). Welfare was reported as an income source by over half the sample (59%).

Psychosocial characteristics of these women are reported in Table 3. About 1 out of every 10 of these women was homeless, that is, reported living in the streets or in a shelter. In addition, although three-quarters (74%) had children, less than one-third (31%) had any children living with them.

As part of the follow-up interview, women were asked about several potential life stresses. Thus, the data regarding life stresses were based only on the follow-up sample of 380 women. A majority of women reported one or more traumatic life stresses including

Table 3. Psycho-Social Characteristics of HAP Women

Living circumstances: 10% homeless

Had children: 73%

Living with children: 31%

Life Stresses and Knowledge of Others with HIV/AIDS:*

Life stresses:	Relative or close friend killed:	68%
	Victim of sexual assault:	47%
	Family member abused by police:	37%
	Relative or close friend died of drug overdose:	51%
	Been in foster care or group home:	19%

Know anyone who has HIV/AIDS:		65%
Number of people you know with HIV/AIDS:		6.0
Know anyone who has died of AIDS:		54%

* This section is based on information collected at the six month follow-up, n=380).

having a relative or close friend who was killed (68%), being the victim of sexual assault (47%) and having a relative or close friend who died of a drug overdose (51%). Women were also asked about whether they knew people who were HIV positive or had AIDS. As can be seen from the table, about two-thirds knew someone with HIV/AIDS and those women who knew someone, knew an average of 6 people. More than half the women (54%) reported knowing at least one person who had died of AIDS. The women were also asked if they were involved in the care of someone with AIDS, and 6% of them responded yes.

In addition to interview data, ethnographic data were collected through the use of life histories and participant observation in the community. Ethnographic findings indicated that many clients had experienced traumatic lives; and that clients may perceive AIDS risk reduction as less critical an issue than other more immediately threatening concerns such as homelessness (Clatts, Beardsley, Deren, & Tortu, 1991).

RESULTS OF THE HAP INTERVENTION

As reported previously (Deren, Tortu, Davis, in press), the women participating in HAP reported substantial reductions in both needle use and sexual risk behaviors from baseline to six-month follow-up. For example, almost one-third of the IDUs (31%) reported no longer injecting at follow-up. In addition, repeated measures analyses comparing baseline and follow-up data indicated reductions in such risk variables as average monthly injection frequency (43 to 13; $p < .001$) and the average monthly number of unprotected sexual acts (37 to 19; $p < .001$). Reductions were reported across all groups of women, those who participated in the standard intervention as well as those participating in the enhanced intervention. This may indicate that risk reduction was occurring throughout the community, and the relatively short term (three-session) enhanced intervention was not sufficient to lead to increases beyond those which were already occurring. The fact that most of these women reported knowing people with HIV and knowing at least one person who had died of AIDS may be related to the level of change reported across individuals participating in the study.

Analyses of the HAP data have been undertaken to identify variables related to greater levels of risk reduction, and demographic, psychological, and life stress data have been assessed; thus far, no consistent relationships have emerged between risk reduction and these variable domains.

The subjects who participated in the group sessions were asked at follow-up whether they had discussed the contents of the groups with others. The overwhelming majority reported that they had discussed the information, with 90% of the women reporting they had discussed it with one or more friends, 87% reported they discussed it with one or more sex partners, 66% reported discussing it with one or more family members and 72% discussed it with one or more "get high" partners, that is, people they used drugs with. Thus it appears that the information in the groups may have filtered out substantially beyond those individuals in actual attendance.

Revised Intervention: CAPA (Cooperative Agreement to Prevent AIDS)

The intervention developed for the newly initiated CAPA project, in East Harlem, was based on experiences in HAP and was designed to use an intensive, multi-modal intervention to lead to more extensive AIDS risk reduction. Table 4 provides a summary of the new CAPA intervention. The social learning model, implemented in the demonstration, practice and reinforcement of health-related skills, was retained as the basis for the intervention. However, the experiences of HAP indicated the need to address issues and teach skills related to problems of primary concern to clients, and not simply AIDS related. The primary rationale is that if individuals learn skills and develop self-efficacy related to health promotion which addresses immediate concerns, this can provide the basis for self-efficacy and the development of skills related to HIV prevention. Thus, the new curriculum has 9 components, and addresses such areas as general health and well-being, accessing social services, and stress management.

The methods used in the group sessions are based on Freire's popular education model, and use games and other participatory exercises to validate clients' abilities and insure their participation in the learning process (Tobkes, Springer, Plaga, Deren, & Tortu,

Table 4. New CAPA Intervention

A. Theoretical Model:

- In a social learning model, curriculum addresses clients' needs and concerns (Health and Nutrition, Accessing Services;   Families, Harm Reduction, Sex and STDs, Stress Management,   Violence and Abuse, HIV/AIDS)

B. Methods:

- Uses educational methods which enhance skills/self-efficacy
- Provides active referrals
- Provides peer models for behavior change

1990). This teaching method encourages persons to develop certain analytical skills and devise their own techniques to address issues related to social and physical wellness. The educational process itself thus becomes a method to enhance self-efficacy. The preliminary development of the application of Popular Education ideas to AIDS prevention efforts was pilot tested in the second year of HAP. A curriculum guide was developed for all 9 components during the start-up phase of the CAPA project.

Another aspect of the revised intervention model addresses clients' needs for access and involvement with health and social service agencies. The project uses a modified case management approach; all clients assigned to the enhanced intervention meet with a referral coordinator for a needs assessment and active referrals. Active referrals include telephoning the referral service and providing an escort to clients, if needed, to assist them in reaching and successfully accessing services. Finally, individuals who participated successfully in HAP, and come from the East Harlem community, have been recruited to co-lead the education groups and serve as escorts to referrals. Thus, models for behavior change are provided so that clients may be more able to identify and model after peers who have incorporated substantial risk reduction in their lives. The extent to which HAP clients reported discussing group contents with peers and friends in the community indicates that reinforcing the utilization of peers as role models may be effective in enhancing behavior changes.

CONCLUSIONS

A summary of the conclusions appears in Table 5. Although research indicates that the high risk women report substantial risk reductions, more extensive efforts to develop interventions which address the multitude of social and economic difficulties experienced by these women is indicated. Although both a Standard and Enhanced intervention led to significant behavior changes, the development and assessment of interventions which maximally affect risk behaviors are needed.

The HAP research indicates that continued efforts are needed to identify the best predictors of risk reduction; further analyses of existing data sets as well as additional research efforts, perhaps incorporating other psychological and contextual variables (e.g., reaction to the level of seroprevalence in the community) should be undertaken.

In addition, for high seroprevalence areas in particular, research to assess the impact of the epidemic itself, and the social consequences of living in a community where there are large numbers of people who are HIV positive and progressing to AIDS, in itself requires further investigation. Efforts to understand and enhance

Table 5. Conclusions

- Female IDUs and sex partners can significantly reduce risk behaviors
- More extensive efforts to identify maximally effective risk reduction interventions are needed
- Addressing clients multiple social and economic needs and concerns appear necessary to fully address and impact on the epidemic. Efforts which just focus on specific needle and sex risk behaviors, although successful, are not likely to be sufficient for extensive long-lasting change.
- Further research on the variables related to risk reduction is needed
- The social and psychological impact of the epidemic, particularly in high seroprevalence communities, should be assessed

skills for coping with this tragedy, particularly for previously traumatized individuals, who are themselves at high risk for becoming HIV positive, are needed. Both qualitative and quantitative studies of the psychological and social impacts of the epidemic, including its impact on risk reduction among high risk individuals is needed.

REFERENCES

Bandura, A. (1977). Social learning theory. Englewood Cliffs, NJ: Prentice-Hall.

Bandura, A. (1987, September). Perceived self-efficacy in the exercise of control over AIDS Infection. Presented at the Conference on Women and AIDS: Promoting Health Behaviors, Bethesda, MD.

Centers for Disease Control, Public Health Service (1992, January). *HIV/AIDS surveillance update*. Atlanta.

Clatts, M., Beardsley, M., Deren, S., & Tortu, S. (1991, October). Economies of scale and the homeless drug injector: Contradictions in AIDS prevention practice–An ethnographic perspective. Presented at the Third Annual National AIDS Demonstration and Research Conference, Washington, DC.

Deren, S. (1989, October). The Harlem AIDS Project: Description and preliminary findings. Presented at the First Annual National AIDS Demonstration and Research Conference, Rockville, MD.

Deren, S., Tortu, S., Davis, W.R. (in press). An AIDS risk reduction project with inner-city women. In T. Squire (Ed.), *Women, Psychology and AIDS*, Sage Publications.

Hartgers, S., Van den Hoek, J.A.R., Coutinho, R.A., & Van Der Pligt, J. (1990, June). Determinants of injecting and sexual risk behavior among HIV-Negative injecting drug users. Presented at the Sixth International Conference on AIDS, San Francisco.

Health Services Administration (HSA /N.Y.C.) (1990, May). HIV infection and IV drug use estimates by neighborhood. New York, NY.

New York City, Office of AIDS Surveillance (1991, January 31). AIDS surveillance update: Fourth quarter 1991 (specific breakdowns were also obtained through personal communication with this office). New York, NY.

Tobkes, C., Springer, E., Plaga, E., Deren, S., & Tortu, S. (1990, August). Adapting AIDS education for active drug using populations. Presented at the IV International Conference on AIDS Education. San Juan.

Characteristics of Female Sexual Partners of Injection Drug Users in Southern Arizona: Implications for Effective HIV Risk Reduction Interventions

Sally J. Stevens, PhD
Julie Reed Erickson, PhD
Antonio L. Estrada, PhD

SUMMARY. Epidemiological data suggest that women who are sexual partners of injection drug users (IDUs) are at increasing risk for HIV (CDC, 1992). This study describes characteristics of 180 female sexual partners (FSPs) living in southern Arizona. These characteristics include ethnicity, age, income source, living arrangement,

Sally J. Stevens is Director of Research, Amity, Inc., 47 E. Pennington, Tucson, AZ 85701. Julie Reed Erickson is Assistant Professor, University of Arizona, College of Medicine, 2501 E. Elm Street, Tucson, AZ 85716. Antonio L. Estrada is Research Coordinator, Latino Health and Mental Health Unit, Mexican American Studies and Research Center, University of Arizona, Douglass Building, Room 315, Tucson, AZ 85721.

This research was supported by the National Institute on Drug Abuse, Community Research Branch; 5 R18DA05748.

[Haworth co-indexing entry note]: "Characteristics of Female Sexual Partners of Injection Drug Users in Southern Arizona: Implications for Effective HIV Risk Reduction Interventions." Stevens, Sally J., Julie Reed Erickson, and Antonio L. Estrada. Co-published simultaneously in *Drugs & Society* (The Haworth Press, Inc.) Vol. 7, No. 3/4, 1993, pp. 129-142; and: *AIDS and Community-Based Drug Intervention Programs: Evaluation and Outreach* (ed: Dennis G. Fisher, and Richard Needle) The Haworth Press, Inc., 1993, pp. 129-142. Multiple copies of this article/chapter may be purchased from The Haworth Document Delivery Center [1-800-3-HAWORTH; 9:00 a.m. - 5:00 p.m. (EST)].

Copyright © 1993 by Taylor & Francis

sexual risk behavior, reasons for sexual risk, and knowledge of AIDS risk and transmission. Data from this study indicate that FSPs vary a great deal on all of these characteristics and thus a single "profile" of FSPs is difficult to conceptualize. Implications of the data suggest that effective interventions for HIV risk reduction for FSPs should be personalized to fit the specific characteristics and needs of the individual.

Epidemiological data suggest that women who are sexual partners of injection drug users (IDUs) are at increasing risk for the human immune-deficiency virus (HIV). In part this is due to the increase in the number of HIV positive individuals who are IDUs. Over the first decade of the acquired immune deficiency syndrome (AIDS) epidemic, national statistics demonstrate a shift in case distribution towards IDUs (Coates et al. 1990). In 1981, 65% of AIDS cases were attributed to male homo-bisexual contact, 11% to intravenous drug use and 0.5% to heterosexual contact. In 1989, male homo-bisexual transmission accounted for 55% of new AIDS cases, intravenous drug use for 23% and heterosexual contact for 5% (Centers for Disease Control, 1990).

These epidemiological data are reflected in the increase in women who are sexual partners of injection drug users (IDUs) who are contracting HIV. Curran et al. (1988) as well as Guinan and Hardy (1987) report unprotected sexual intercourse with an infected male IDU accounts for over 67% of heterosexually acquired AIDS cases in women. By the end of 1991 a total of 4,484 cases of AIDS had been reported by women whose primary risk factor was sexual contact with a male IDU (Centers for Disease Control, 1992). One out of every five women with AIDS is a female sexual partner (FSP) of an IDU, the majority representing minority women. Fifty percent of FSPs with AIDS are Black, 30% are Hispanic, 19% are White, and 1% of FSPs are Native American or Asian.

Research regarding HIV risk behaviors exhibited by FSPs has been examined. Studies conducted in several cities in the United States demonstrate lack of condom use by FSPs. In a study conducted in Miami, Florida, 96% of crack cocaine using women and 90% of non-crack cocaine using women reported having sex with one or more IDUs. When questioned at baseline regarding condom use in the previous 6 months, both crack cocaine users and non users reported that they used condoms less than half the time (McCoy, Miles & Inciardi, 1992). In Long Beach, California, 94.9% of FSPs reported engaging in unprotected vaginal inter-course and 6.6% reported unprotected anal intercourse (Corby, Wo-litski, Thornton-Johnson & Tanner 1991). In a nationwide study of FSPs only 10% reported consistent condom use (Weissman & National AIDS Research Consortium, 1991).

Similar sexual risk behavior data is reported from IDUs who were questioned about their sexual practices with FSPs during the previous 6 month period. In a nationwide study of more than 12,500 male IDUs, 81% reported engaging in vaginal intercourse. Of this 81% only 30% reported ever using a condom. Furthermore, 16% of the 12,500 IDUs reported anal intercourse in the previous 6 months. Of this 16% only 22% reported ever using a condom (Centers for Disease Control, 1990).

While these data demonstrate high levels of sexual risk behavior by FSPs, existing data also suggest that FSPs demonstrate some knowledge of how HIV is transmitted and prevented. In the study by Corby et al. (1991), 137 FSPs in Long Beach, California an-swered questions reflecting their knowledge of HIV transmission and prevention. All but one woman knew that HIV could be trans-mitted by sharing injection equipment and that persons with AIDS could transmit the disease sexually. Eighty-two percent were also aware that latex condoms protected against sexual transmission of HIV. In a national study of FSPs AIDS knowledge was also rela-tively high. Fifty-five percent of FSPs correctly answered 12 or more items on a 15 item HIV knowledge test (Weissman & National AIDS Research Consortium, 1991).

Data on at-risk groups and trends in HIV infection in southern Arizona reflect data reported in other cities of the United States. Epide-miological data from southern Arizona's Pima County (1983-1992) indicate that up to 17% of AIDS cases can be attributed to injection drug use. Up to twenty-one percent of HIV asymptomatic cases can be attributed to injection drug use. The percent of female AIDS cases is 6% and the percent of female HIV asymptomatic cases is 8%. These data indicate a trend in the increase in HIV infection for IDUs and females. Furthermore, an increase in the percent of mino-rities, particularly Hispanics, who have become infected has been documented. AIDS cases in Pima County by ethnicity (1983-1992) include 79% White, 6% Black, 13% Hispanic and 1% Native American. HIV asymptomatic cases include 64% White, 6% Black, 19% Hispanic and 2% Native American (Pima County Health Department, 1992).

Erickson, Estrada and Stevens (1990) reported that FSPs in southern Arizona exhibit high sexual risk behavior. Fifty-five percent of the FSPs had more than one sexual partner in the previous six month period and 45% had multiple sexual partners. Condom use was low for FSPs. Those with a single sexual partner reported using condoms between never and less than half the time while those with multiple sexual partners reported using condoms less than half the time. Most women used noninjectable drugs, which Coates et al. (1990) suggest increases the risk of acquiring HIV through sexual transmission.

Knowledge of AIDS transmission and prevention varied for FSPs in southern Arizona. Some FSPs exhibited excellent knowledge of AIDS transmission and prevention on a 16 item questionnaire. The mean score was 12.6 (SD = 2.18) with a range of 7-16 correct responses. Several of the items that relate directly to female partner risk for AIDS had a high percent of incorrect responses. The majority of women answered incorrectly to the items "Anyone having sex with only one other person cannot get the AIDS virus" (81% incorrect) and "A person can avoid getting the AIDS virus by just having oral sex" (75% incorrect). Other items related to sexual transmission of AIDS had a low percent of incorrect responses. These items were "using a latex condom is an effective way to keep from getting the AIDS virus" (14% incorrect), "A person can get the AIDS virus from having sex with a man who has had sex with another man" (4% incorrect), "A person can get the AIDS virus from having unprotected sex with a person who has AIDS" (3% incorrect), and "A woman with the AIDS virus can give her unborn child AIDS" (3% incorrect) (Erickson, Estrada & Stevens, 1990).

Clearly, there are similarities between southern Arizona and other areas of the country in terms of data supporting the increase in HIV infection for women and minorities as well as similarities in data on HIV risks and knowledge of AIDS transmission reported by FSPs. FSPs exhibit high risk sexual behaviors while demonstrating a moderate to high level of knowledge concerning HIV transmission and prevention. While this information helps FSP advocates to understand that FSPs are at increasing risk and why they are at increasing risk, these data do not tell us much about how one can effectively intervene so that HIV risk reduction can be successfully obtained.

To develop an effective intervention aimed at HIV risk reduction for FSPs, information beyond their risk behaviors and knowledge of HIV is needed. Additional information such as ethnicity, age, income source, living arrangements, and reasons for sexual risks might help to illuminate characteristics that are crucial to the design of an effective intervention.

In southern Arizona, work toward the understanding of characteristics of sexual partners has been underway since April, 1989. The Community Outreach Project on AIDS in Southern Arizona (COPASA) is a HIV research and intervention project funded by the National Institute of Drug Abuse, Community Research Branch. The specific aims of COPASA are to: (a) document AIDS risk behaviors among IDUs and sexual partners of IDUs, especially among ethnic minorities; and (b) intervene to reduce AIDS risk. In COPASA, sexual partners include adult men and women who have had sex with an IDU but have not injected drugs in the last six months.

The purpose of this paper is to describe characteristics among FSPs enrolled in COPASA in an effort to help create an effective intervention strategy.

METHODS

All women meeting criteria as a sexual partner were invited to participate in COPASA. Outreach workers recruited FSPs at project sites in a large city, small community and Native American nation in southern Arizona. Eighty-five percent of the FSPs were recruited through street outreach. Fifteen percent were inmates who were recruited through the county jail.

Data describing female sexual partners for this paper were gathered at enrollment into COPASA. Information on ethnicity, age, income source, living arrangements, sexual risk behaviors, reasons for sexual risk behaviors, and knowledge of AIDS risk and transmission were collected using the AIDS Initial Assessment (AIA) developed by the National Institute on Drug Abuse. The AIA is a 200 item questionnaire administered by a trained interviewer in a private, individual session. Support for reliability and validity of the AIA in measuring AIDS risk exist (Myers, Snyderm, Bryant & Young, 1990).

Data were analyzed using the Statistical Package for the Social Sciences (SPSS, 1988). Characteristics of this convenience sample were analyzed using descriptive statistics.

RESULTS

Sample Characteristics. One hundred and eighty female sexual partners were enrolled in COPASA. In self reports of their ethnic group 16.1% were White, 32.2% were Hispanic, 39.4% were Native American, 10.6% were Black, and 1.1% were Asian (Table 1).

The average age of the women was 30.06 years (*SD* 9.058) with a range of 18-62 years. White women were older at 34.03 years than Hispanic ($\overline{X}$ = 29.34) Native American ($\overline{X}$ = 29.54) and Black ($\overline{X}$ = 28.42) women (Table 2).

The major income source in the previous 6 months reported by the FSPs was welfare (40.6%). Welfare was followed in order by job (27.2%), spouse/sexual partner (7.8%), family member (6.1%), illegal activity (6.1%), other (2.8%), disability (2.2%), unemployed (1.7%), friends (1.1%), and alimony (.6%). Living arrangements varied for the FSPs with many participants reporting that they lived with their spouse or sexual partner (29.6%) (Table 3). Some partici-

Ethnicity	Frequency	% of Total Sample
White	29	16.2
Hispanic	58	32.4
Native American	71	39.7
Black	19	10.6
Asian	2	1.1

Table 1.   Ethnicity of Female Sexual Partners

	Mean	Standard Deviation
Current Age (N=180)	30.06	9.06
White	34.03	9.89
Hispanic	29.34	8.09
Native American	29.54	8.18
Black	28.42	12.11

Table 2. Age by Ethnicity of Female Sexual Partners

Source of Income	% of Total Sample
Welfare	40.6
Job	27.2
Spouse/Partner	7.8
Family Member	6.1
Illegal Activity	6.1
Other	2.8
Disability	2.2
Unemployment	1.7
Friends	1.1
Alimony	.6
Living Arrangement	**% of Total**
Sexual Partner	29.6
Adult Relatives	17.9
Parents	14.1
Alone	10.7
Friends	10.7
Other	16.9

Table 3. Income Source and Living Arrangements for Female Sexual Partners

pants lived with adult relatives (17.9%), some lived with parents (14.1%), some lived alone (10.7%), some lived with friends (10.7%), and 16.9% reported living in an "other" situation.

The number of sexual partners is a risk factor in HIV transmission. Of the 177 FSPs who responded to questions regarding the number of sexual partners 97 (54.8%) reported having a single sexual partner and 80 (45.2%) reported having multiple sexual partners. Among the racial groups, differences existed in terms of the number reporting single or multiple sexual partners. The majority of Hispanic and Native American women reported a single partner while most White and Black women reported multiple sexual partners (Table 4).

Frequency of condom use was examined. On a scale of 0 (never use condoms) to 4 (always use condoms), those having a single partner had a mean of 0.54, indicating they used condoms between never and less than half the time. FSPs of all ethnic groups who had a single sexual partner reported similar condom use. Women with multiple partners used condoms on the average less than half the time ($\overline{X} = .92$). Black women with multiple sexual partners wore condoms more frequently ($\overline{X} = 1.80$) than did Hispanic ($\overline{X} = .79$), Native American ($\overline{X} = .46$), or White ($\overline{X} = 1.30$) women (Table 5).

In an earlier analysis conducted by Erickson, Estrada and Stevens (1990) on 122 FSPs, ninety-seven percent of female partners with male contacts reported vaginal intercourse without the use of a condom at least once in the previous six months. On a scale of 0

Racial Ethnic Group	Single		Multiple	
	n	% of group	n	% of group
Total	97	54.8	80	45.2
Black	9	47.4	10	52.6
Hispanic	34	58.6	24	41.4
Native American	45	63.3	26	36.6
White	9	31.0	20	69.0

Table 4.   Number of Sexual Partners in the Previous Six Months

Numbers of Partners	Mean	Standard Deviation
Single (n=94)	.54	1.11
Black	.55	.72
Hispanic	.38	.92
Native American	.62	1.13
White	.50	1.33
Multiple (n=82)	.92	1.39
Black	1.80	1.62
Hispanic	.79	1.35
Native American	.46	1.10
White	1.30	1.49

Table 5. Frequency of Condom Use by Female Sexual Partners in the Previous Six Months

Response: 0 = never

1 = less than half the time

2 = about half the time

3 = more than half the time

4 = always

(never) to 6 (more than four times a day), vaginal intercourse with a condom occurred between 1-6 times per week ($\overline{X}$ = 2.57). Forty-seven percent reported oral sex with a male contact in the previous six months. On the same scale of 0-6 for frequency, oral sex without condoms occurred less than 4 times per month ($\overline{X}$ = 1.06). Anal intercourse without the use of a condom occurred at least once in the previous six months for 16% of the women. On the average using the same frequency scale, anal intercourse without a condom took place much less than 4 times per month ($\overline{X}$ = 0.24)

Virtually all the 180 FSPs reported that they did not always use condoms. They were then asked, "Why don't you use condoms?" (Table 6). Of these women, 126 responded to the question. Their responses were categorized into partner-related and self-related reasons. "My partner does not like to use condoms" was the most

Category	Frequency	% of Total
Category: Partner Related		
Partner not like to use	43	34.1
Fear of partner	14	11.1
Afraid of getting hurt	2	1.6
Partner free of AIDS	2	1.6
Accuse partner of AIDS	2	1.6
Can't get AIDS	1	0.8
Category: Self Related		
Not like to use	35	27.8
Want baby	11	8.7
Too high	10	7.9
Uneasy using condom	5	4.0
Can't give AIDS	1	0.8
Total Responses	126	100%

Table 6.   Categories and Frequencies of Response to "Why Don't You Always Use a Condom?"   ($\underline{n}$=126)

frequent response (34.1%). "I don't like to use condoms" was the next most frequent response (27.8%). Other reasons given in the partner related category were fear of the partner including fear of getting hurt, feelings that the partner did not have AIDS, not wanting to accuse the partner of having AIDS and personal feeling that she could not get AIDS. Other reasons given in the self category were wanting to have a baby, being uneasy about condom use, being too high to use condoms and a feeling that she could not give AIDS to anyone.

Knowledge of AIDS risk and transmission was assessed using a 16 item true-false questionnaire (Table 7). For all female sexual partners, the average number of correct responses was 12.89 (*SD* 2.06) with a range of 7-16 correct responses. Although ethnic differences in terms of the number of correct responses were slight, differences in correct answers for various questions was extreme. Some of the women knew

Group	Mean	Standard Deviation
Total Sample	12.9	2.06
Black	14.0	1.36
Hispanic	12.2	2.53
Native American	12.8	1.80
White	13.4	1.91

Table 7a. Knowledge of AIDS Risk and Transmission Among Female Sexual Partners: Knowledge scores

Response range: 0 = none correct to 16 = all correct

Items	% Incorrect Response
Can't get AIDS if only 1 partner	73.3
Can't get AIDS with oral sex	77.2
Can't get AIDS with latex condom	15.6
Woman with AIDS can give to child	1.7
Can get AIDS from bisexual	3.9
Can't get AIDS with unprotected sex with AIDS person	1.7

Table 7b. Knowledge of AIDS Risk and Transmission Among Female Sexual Partners. Incorrect responses to specific items

very little about HIV transmission, scoring 7 on the forced choiced 16 item questionnaire. A score of 7 reflects less than what someone might score by chance. Other women exhibited a great deal of knowledge regarding HIV transmission answering all 16 items correctly.

DISCUSSION

In examining characteristics of FSPs one can conclude that there is wide variation in the women that this term attempts to describe. In southern Arizona, FSPs are of several ethnic groups. The age range of the women is very wide (18 to 62 years) with the mean age of ethnic groups reflecting a great deal of variation as well ($\overline{X}$ = 28.42 for Black women compared with $\overline{X}$ = 34.03 for White women). Although 40.6% of the FSPs report welfare as their main income source, 9 other major sources of income were reported. Self reports on living arrangements also demonstrate wide variation in the lives of FSPs in southern Arizona. A relatively even spread of 5 of the 6 living situations was documented with "living with spouse/sexual partner" being the living situation to be reported most frequently (29.6%).

The research suggests that there is variation in FSPs' knowledge of AIDS risk and transmission. While mean scores did not vary for ethnic groups the range of correct response was from 43.7% correct to 100% correct. In examining which questions were answered incorrectly it appears that some FSPs are not aware of the link between sex and HIV. Furthermore, for those women who do understand the link between sex and AIDS, knowledge does not translate into behaviors such as using condoms when engaging in sex with an IDU.

When one examines variables on risk of contracting HIV and reasons that FSPs give for taking those risks, the data reflect wide variation. The number of sexual partners that FSP reports is evenly split with 53.4% reporting a single sexual partner and 46.6% reporting multiple sexual partners. While condom use is low for all FSPs, reasons for not using condoms is also split with 50.8% reporting that the reason is "partner related" while 49.2% reporting the reason for not using condoms was "self related."

In observing these differences and variations in characteristics of FSPs in southern Arizona it seems clear that a single "profile" of a FSP would be difficult, if not impossible, to develop. Barriers to condom use and changing behavior to lower the risk for contracting HIV may be tangled within a multitude of personal characteristics and the specific situation of each woman.

As FSP advocates work to develop effective interventions the data presented here indicate that generic "one intervention for all FSPs" is not appropriate. On the contrary, an effective intervention aimed at lowering HIV risk behaviors must untangle the web of each woman's life. Erickson, Estrada, and Stevens (1990) and Stevens, DeGroff and Ruiz (1992) found that FSPs identify their concern of becoming HIV infected as "low" when comparing it to other concerns such as food, clothing, shelter for themselves and their children, concern for obtaining non-injectable drugs such as crack cocaine, and concern about being arrested.

FSP advocates working at the COPASA project in southern Arizona redesigned their intervention for FSPs as data from the FSP component increased their understanding of (a) the characteristics of FSPs, (b) FSPs' understanding of HIV transmission, (c) exhibited risk behaviors of FSPs.

The COPASA project offers a "standardized intervention" that includes the traditional components of HIV prevention information, condom skill acquisition and HIV testing. COPASA also offers an enhanced intervention. Included in the enhanced intervention is a discussion of the FSPs' various psycho-social factors related to her immediate life situation. This part of the intervention helps the FSP advocate to understand the uniqueness of the participant's life and her specific situation. The FSP advocate is then able to offer suggestions to various problems as well as offer appropriate social service referrals.

The FSP advocate discusses with the FSP the link between sex and AIDS. A personalized goal setting component is then facilitated. Together the FSP advocate and FSP outline reasonable and achievable goals aimed at lowering her risk of contracting HIV. These goals may differ dramatically from participant to participant. In concluding the session the FSP advocate clarifies that the COPASA site can always be used as a resource: for social service information and referrals, condoms, telephone, etc.

Follow-up sessions reviewing the personalized HIV risk reduction goals are facilitated by the FSP advocate every six to eight weeks for a six-month period. Because many women may have difficulty getting to the COPASA site, these sessions are designed to be facilitated anywhere in the community (COPASA site, participant's home, park, restaurant, etc.). If the risk reduction goals have been successfully achieved, new goals are developed. If the risk reduction goals have not been achieved, barriers to achieving the goals are discussed. The goals are then adjusted as appropriate to the woman's specific situation.

Data from past projects reflect some success with interventions that address risk reduction; however, those successes are, at times, minimal. It is necessary to examine not only the interventions, but also the characteristics of the women for whom the interventions were and were not successful. Although a "single profile" of a FSP for the COPASA sample appears impossible to develop, perhaps conducting a cluster analysis of cases might provide enlightening information. Furthermore, new research based on previous findings is crucial in identifying which interventions and what factors within the intervention allow for HIV risk reduction behavior change.

REFERENCES

Centers for Disease Control. (1992, January). *HIV/AIDS Surveillance Report.*

Centers for Disease Control. (1990). Risk behaviors for HIV transmission among intravenous drug users not in drug treatment–United States, 1987-1989. *Morbidity & Mortality Weekly Report, 39*, 273-276.

Centers for Disease Control. (1990). *HIV/AIDS surveillance: U.S. AIDS cases reported through December 1989.* Atlanta, GA.

Coates, T., Des Jarlais, D., Miller, H., Moses, L., Turner, C., & Worth, D. (1990). The AIDS epidemic in the second decade. In H. Miller, C. Turner & L. Moses (Eds.), *AIDS: The Second decade.* Washington, DC: National Academy Press.

Corby, N. H., Wolitski, R. J., Thornton-Johnson, S., and Tanner, W. M. (1991). Aids knowledge, perception of risk, and behaviors among female sex partners of injection drug users. *AIDS Education and Prevention, 3*, 353-366.

Curran, J., Jaffe, H., Hardy, A., Morgan, W., Selik, R., & Dondero, T. (1988). Epidemiology of HIV infection and AIDS in the United States. *Science, 239*, 610-616.

Erickson, J. R., Estrada, A. L., Stevens, S. J. (1990). *Risk for AIDS among female sexual partners of IVDU's.* Presented at the 118th Annual Meeting of the American Public Health Association, New York, NY.

Guinan, M. & Hardy, A. (1987). Epidemiology of AIDS in women in the United States: 1981-1986. *Journal of the American Medical Association, 257*, 2039-2042.

McCoy, H. V., Miles, C., Inciardi, J. (1991). *Survival sex: Inner-city women and crack cocaine.* Presented at the Third Annual National AIDS Demonstration Research Meeting, Washington, DC.

Myers, M., Snyder, F., Bryant, E., & Young, P. (in press). Report on the reliability of the AIDS Initial Assessment. Presented at the First Annual National AIDS Demonstration Research Meeting (NIDA Research Monograph).

Pima County Health Department. (1992, February). *AIDS Surveillance Report.*

SPSS. (1988). *SPSS-X User's Guide (3rd ed.).* Chicago: SPSS, Inc.

Stevens, S. J., DeGroff, A., Ruiz, D. (1992). Focus group data from crack cocaine using women. Unpublished report, Tucson and Phoenix, AZ.

Weissman, G. & National AIDS Research Consortium. (1991). AIDS prevention for women at risk: Experience from a national research demonstration program. *Journal of Primary Prevention, 12*, 49-63.

An Emerging Public Health Model for Reducing AIDS-Related Risk Behavior Among Injecting Drug Users and Their Sexual Partners

Clyde B. McCoy, PhD
James E. Rivers, PhD
Elizabeth L. Khoury, RN, MA

SUMMARY. An efficient and cost-effective public health model for reducing AIDS-related risk behavior among injecting drug users and their sexual partners is emerging from data obtained from NIDA's multi-site National AIDS Demonstration Research (NADR) project. Long-term (18-month post-intervention) follow-up data from the Miami site demonstrate the durability of substantial risk reduction among project participants, related to both drug use and sexual behavior. Public health, drug treatment, and other health care providers should be aware of successful outreach intervention strategies and incorporate them into state and local AIDS prevention programs targeting out-of-treatment drug users and their sexual partners.

Clyde B. McCoy, James E. Rivers, and Elizabeth L. Khoury are affiliated with the Comprehensive Drug Research Center, University of Miami, 1400 N.W. 10th Avenue, Suite 210, Miami, FL 33136.

[Haworth co-indexing entry note]: "An Emerging Public Health Model for Reducing AIDS-Related Risk Behavior Among Injecting Drug Users and Their Sexual Partners." McCoy, Clyde B., James E. Rivers, and Elizabeth L. Khoury. Co-published simultaneously in *Drugs & Society* (The Haworth Press, Inc.) Vol. 7, No. 3/4, 1993, pp. 143-159; and: *AIDS and Community-Based Drug Intervention Programs: Evaluation and Outreach* (ed: Dennis G. Fisher, and Richard Needle) The Haworth Press, Inc., 1993, pp. 143-159. Multiple copies of this article/chapter may be purchased from The Haworth Document Delivery Center [1-800-3-HAWORTH; 9:00 a.m. - 5:00 p.m. (EST)].

Copyright © 1993 by Taylor & Francis

The first responses to the Acquired Immune Deficiency Syndrome (AIDS) epidemic, understandably, were dominated by hastily-mounted efforts to inform specific populations–initially, only homosexual, later, injection drug users (IDUs), much later, sexual partners of IDUs–that were at risk. The focus was upon information to raise awareness, the emphasis was upon saturation implementation (Coyle, Boruch, & Turner, 1991). The immediacy of the need to alert potential victims overshadowed any major attention to such "ideal" characteristics of prevention programs as foundation of tested theory (or at least well-conceived, experience-based rationale) feasibility, acceptability, adaptability, exportability, generalizability to other populations, and strong implementation in order to achieve durable effects and to be evaluated (Botvin, 1988).

More recently, significant attention and resources have begun to be directed to the development of knowledge and techniques that will help to inspire or induce changes in sexual and drug-using behaviors which pose risks for Human Immunodeficiency Virus (HIV) infection. Most of these efforts are in relatively early stages (Turner, Miller, & Moses, 1989), but a general finding seems to already be clear: The advances made in our general understanding of health-related behaviors (Clark, 1987; Strecher, Devellis, Becker, & Rosenstock, 1986) provide a useful, but incomplete, foundation for designing and implementing education, prevention, or more active intervention programs for the specific high-risk populations of injection drug users and their sexual partners.

Only the most naive would ever think that motivating IDUs to change their HIV risk-associated drug-using and sexual behaviors would be a simple task. These are learned and often internalized behaviors–strengthened by time and repetition–which may define a preferred lifestyle, which may be driven by physiological as well as psychological addiction, and which may be perceived by the at-risk individuals to be essential to the maintenance of valued personal and sexual relationships. From the more vital perspectives of societal values and their reflection in public policy, there is a prevalent perception that IDUs–by "nature" and definition–are self-destructive and are incapable of sustaining long-term behavioral change.

Yet, a number of studies provide accumulating evidence that IDUs will modify their behavior to reduce their risk of contracting

AIDS. The earliest risk reduction studies conducted among New York City IDUs–both in treatment and out–reported that many sought sterile injection equipment, reduced the number of individuals with whom they shared needles, and reduced or ceased drug injection (Des Jarlais, Friedman, & Hopkins, 1985; Friedman, Des Jarlais, & Sotheran, 1986; Selwyn, Feiner, Cox, Lipshutz, & Cohen, 1987; Sotheran, 1986). Two San Francisco community outreach demonstration projects reported that many IDUs had adopted the use of bleach–small bottles of which were distributed by the projects–to sterilize their injection equipment (Moss, & Chaisson, 1988; Watters, 1987). Reductions in the AIDS-related sexual risk behavior of IDUs have been reported as well, albeit of lesser magnitude than reductions reported for drug-injection-associated risk behaviors (Donoghoe, Stimson, & Dolan, 1989; Turner et al., 1989; Van den Hoak, 1990). These and similar evaluation reports from even the early demonstration efforts provided limited specific knowledge but–equally important at this juncture–an empirical basis for hope regarding the potential for success of behavioral interventions to prevent the spread of HIV infection (Turner et al., 1989).

The informed consensus was that demonstration projects and associated evaluation research were crucial if more effective risk-reduction programs were to be developed and resources and services appropriately allocated. Consequently, the National Institute on Drug Abuse (NIDA) initiated in 1987 the multi-site National AIDS Demonstration Research (NADR) project to develop and to test the efficacy of various HIV-related behavioral risk-reduction intervention models.

THE NATIONAL AIDS DEMONSTRATION RESEARCH PROJECT

The NADR project was designed to provide rapid response to the critical need for detailed knowledge of how to achieve optimum effectiveness in reducing HIV-related risk behaviors among IDUs utilizing minimal resources and brief interventions. NIDA chose the mechanism of a coordinated multi-site network of demonstration prevention/intervention research projects. The initial round of awards was granted to localities known to have high AIDS prevalence rates. The NADR project was directed mainly at IDUs who were not currently in drug treatment (estimated at the time to be approximately 85% of the total target population) and the sexual partners of IDUs. Its goal was to implement and evaluate applied intervention strategies for achieving and maintaining reductions in HIV-related sexual and drug-using risk behavior among these populations. Additional project objectives were to conduct exploratory research on sexual and drug use behaviors associated with increased risk of HIV infection (Weddington et al., 1990).

By 1989, NADR projects were operational at 41 sites throughout the United States and Puerto Rico. Some of the many common features of the projects included: (1) the use of outreach workers/recruiters who frequently were ex-addicts themselves and who were indigenous to the community to be targeted; (2) project participation eligibility criteria of (a) drug injection during the prior six months, and (b) no participation in a formal drug treatment program in the prior 30 days, or (c) being or having been the sexual partner of an IDU; (3) using trained interviewers to collect baseline data on risk behavior, relevant socio-demographic information, and knowledge about AIDS using the standardized AIDS Initial Assessment (AIA) questionnaire; (4) the opportunity (in most programs) to have a blood test to determine the presence of antibodies to HIV, accompanied by appropriate pre- and post-test counseling; (5) administration of either a brief "standard" or a more complex "enhanced" risk reduction regime; and (6) repeat participant interviews and counseling at subsequent six-month intervals, using a standardized AIDS follow-up Assessment (AFA) questionnaire to determine changes in AIDS-related risk behaviors. (Seronegatives were again given a chance to be tested and appropriately informed and counseled.)

While all programs encouraged cessation of injected drug use, prudence dictated a working assumption that this would not be an immediate or uniform outcome. Therefore, the interventions also promoted such safer injection practices as eliminating needle sharing, using sterile injection equipment, and cleaning needles and syringes with bleach when sterile equipment was not available. Abstinence being neither a realistic nor psychosocially preferred goal, the projects universally encouraged safer sexual practices, such as reducing the number of sexual partners, avoiding IDU sexual partners, and using condoms for every sexual encounter. Many of the intervention project sites distributed condoms and/or bleach to study participants.

In contrast to the commonalities outlined above, there were numerous and potentially significant differences among demonstration sites in: (a) the rigor of research designs; (b) the fidelity of implementations to descriptions; (c) the recruitment/sampling strategies used; (d) the enthusiasm with which HIV testing was promoted (and the corresponding completeness of seroincidence and seroconversion data from that site); and (e) the allocation of resources and development of skills/techniques to re-interview and re-test project enrollees six months post-enrollment.

Some NADR projects which were funded from later review cycles are ongoing. A recent analysis of six-month follow-up data from the first six programs funded under this initiative has been completed (Kroliczak & Orange, 1992). In the dissemination of these results, some of the projects were singled out as replicable models of effective outreach-based interventions designed to reduce AIDS-related risk behavior among IDUs and their sexual partners. The intervention model used by the Miami NADR project has been published by the research team, not only to inform the scientific community, but also (in book form) to educate and stimulate discussion in the public arena (Chitwood et al., 1991).

Data from the Miami NADR project are presented and discussed in this paper to provide some of the first answers to the often-asked questions regarding the durability of the observed short-term behavior changes. The specifics of the Miami intervention are briefly described, emphasizing recruitment, intervention, and follow-up techniques and procedures. Finally, the importance of the NADR project (and its successor, the Cooperative Agreement Risk Evaluation (CARE) project) is discussed from a public policy perspective. It is suggested that these projects really are emergent public health models–practical, effective, and efficient alternative paradigms for urban communities internationally–for intervening with IDUs and their sexual partners to retard the transmission of AIDS.

Effective public health action must be based on accurate knowledge of the cause and distribution of health problems and of effective interventions. Despite much progress, for many public health problems the knowledge base, including knowledge about the effectiveness of specific interventions, is inadequate.

DURABILITY OF CHANGES: DATA FROM THE MIAMI NADR PROJECT

Maintenance of behavioral change over time is an issue of paramount importance in AIDS prevention because reverting to previously high levels of risk behavior negates the effectiveness of the intervention program. Because the Miami NADR project was one of the first sites to begin recruitment, it had the opportunity to capture follow-up data at *three* six-month follow-up intervals. This allowed us to begin to answer questions which are crucial to the continuation of the research program and to the prospect that the models developed from it could be adopted as integral components of a broader public health strategy. The ultimate test of the effectiveness of risk reduction intervention programs concerns the extent to which positive behavior changes can be sustained over a long period of time.

The study population for this analysis consists of IDUs who completed three follow-up interviews, providing data on levels of risk behavior for a period of eighteen months after participation in the intervention program. The majority of participants in the baseline sample of IDUs were male (75%) and African-American (71%). Among sexual partners the majority were female (70%) and African-American (76%) (Table 1).

Data are presented at four points in time: (a) baseline, reflecting behavior during the six months prior to participation in the intervention program; and from follow-up intervals (b) six-months, (c) 12-months, and (d) 18-months post-enrollment.

Figure 1 depicts a decline in average usage frequency of the drugs most commonly used (injected and non-injected) by the IDU study participants (not including sexual partners). The most common baseline drug/method of administration combination–injected cocaine-declined at each follow-up point. The frequency of use of injected heroin, injected speedball and non-injected crack also declined from baseline levels, although not as dramatically.

Table 1. Baseline Demographic Characteristics

Characteristic	Miami Street Outreach IDUs		Miami Street Outreach Sex Partners	
	N = 1020		N = 337	
Gender	n	%	n	%
Male	762	74.8	101	30.0
Female	257	25.2	235	69.7
Race				
Black	721	70.8	256	76.0
White	180	17.7	28	8.3
Hispanic	109	10.7	52	15.4
Other	8	.8	1	.3
Age				
18-25	86	8.4	83	24.6
26-35	485	47.6	169	50.1
36-45	374	36.7	67	19.9
46-62	73	7.2	18	5.3

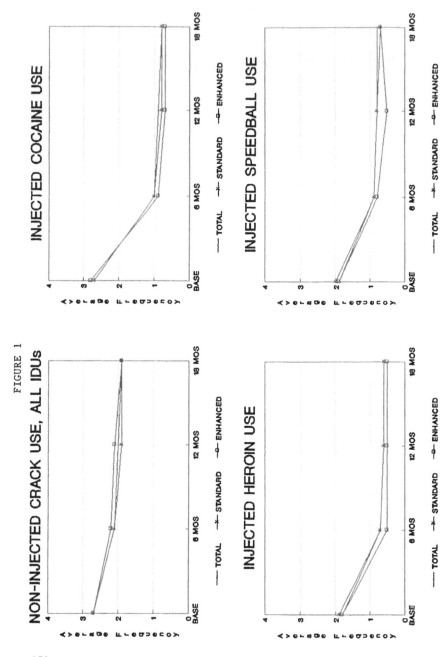

FIGURE 1

A composite measure of needle-associated risk behavior was created by combining three variables: (a) use of rented or borrowed needles, (b) use of non-sterile or uncleaned needles, and (c) sharing with one or more individuals (McCoy, & Khoury, 1990; Snyder, Sowder, & Young, 1989). This index ranks risk on a scale from 0 (no risk) to 11 (highest risk). Figure 2 reflects a decrease in average needle-use-associated risk of IDU study participants at the first follow-up and a maintenance of the lower index results at 12 and 18 month follow-up points. While the frequency of shooting up alone (no needle sharing) increased moderately as compared to baseline data, the frequency of cleaning used needles with bleach increased more dramatically at subsequent follow-up intervals.

A composite measure of sexual risk behavior also was created by combining three pertinent variables; this index was designed to assess the average level of sexually-associated risk of male and female IDUs *and sexual partners*. Risk scores were assigned to three types of sexual practices (vaginal, oral and vaginal sex combined, and anal sex) according to whether or not condoms were used. Number of IDU sexual partners was also incorporated into this index. The lowest risk level (on a scale of 1 to 18) was for an individual with no IDU sexual partners, engaging in vaginal sex with a condom; the highest was for an individual with two or more IDU partners, engaging in anal sex with no condom use (Snyder et al., 1989; McCoy & Khoury, 1990).

As shown in Figure 3, the level of risk declined and was maintained at 12 and 18 month follow-up points for all segments of the study population. Also, lower sexual risk index score averages were derived for female IDUs than for male IDUs and sexual partners.

THE MIAMI OUTREACH MODEL

The Miami NADR project implemented one of the more comprehensive model designs and was either the leading or participating site in numerous supplemental or corollary projects. This discussion of the Miami outreach model focuses on three primary issues: (a) ecological issues such as racial/ethnic differences due to the variety of cultures in Miami; (b) recruitment and follow-up

FIGURE 2

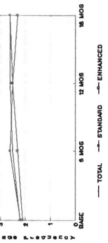

NO NEEDLE SHARING

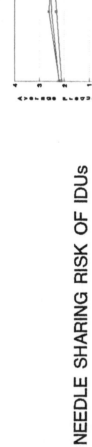

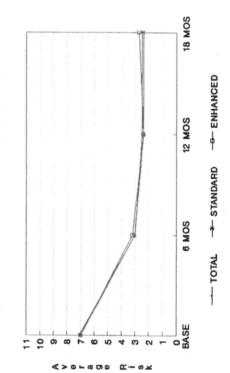

NEEDLE SHARING RISK OF IDUs

NEEDLE CLEANING WITH BLEACH

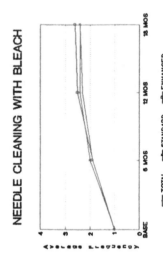

152

FIGURE 3

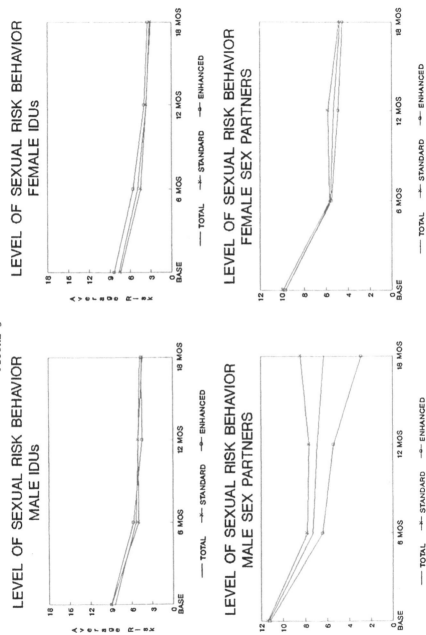

of study participants; and (c) how outreach in itself can be an agent for change.

Ecological Issues

In order to efficiently recruit and interact with potential study participants, the Miami outreach model focused initially on the identification of neighborhoods where the prevalence of drug abuse was particularly high. Through a technique known as geocoding, data obtained from the criminal justice system on arrests for drug-related crimes was computerized and mapped, producing a visual picture of neighborhoods where substantial numbers of IDUs could be located (McCoy, Rivers & Khoury, 1991).

In addition, the research team collaborated with ethnographers who had extensive experience and contacts in the Miami drug use scene and who were able to provide firsthand accounts of procedures in local shooting galleries and crack houses. Data gained from the ethnography studies accentuated the importance of hiring outreach workers similar in gender and ethnicity to the targeted subgroups and indigenous to the neighborhoods selected as recruitment sites. Ethnographic information also suggested the advisability of providing specialized interventions to specific subgroups such as female sexual partners, Hispanics, and participants whose HIV antibody test was positive.

A risk reduction pamphlet promoting needle cleansing and safer sexual behavior was produced in a colorful comic book format for distribution to study participants and potential participants. The pamphlet presented a soap opera vignette of a young inner city woman taking greater control of her life and was pretested in the target community for accuracy of street language and images (McCoy, & Khoury, 1992).

Recruitment and Follow-Up

Indigenous outreach workers, usually former drug users with contacts and credibility in their local neighborhoods, approached potential participants in street settings, such as parks, housing projects, and playgrounds to encourage them to enroll in the intervention program.

Individuals meeting the eligibility requirements were referred to the program's Assessment Center, easily reached from the target communities and located near the county hospital where the majority of the target population received their primary medical care.

An initial pre-test counseling session supplied information on the Enzyme-linked Immunosorbent Assay and Western Blot blood tests. In addition, it provided a supportive setting in which the study participant could decide whether to be tested. After informed consent to participate in the study was given, blood was drawn to obtain a baseline determination of HIV antibody status. Following the blood test, a detailed interview, using the standard AIDS Initial Assessment (AIA) questionnaire, was administered by trained interviewers to assess AIDS-related drug and sexual risk behavior.

After completing the AIA, study participants were randomized into a standard or an enhanced intervention group. Standard intervention participants returned two weeks after their initial assessment to receive post-test counseling and the results of their HIV antibody test. Following Center for Disease Control protocols and NIDA guidelines, post-test counseling included information on the meaning of HIV test results, modes of HIV transmission, and a thorough discussion of risk reduction strategies. A packet of brochures was also given to each standard intervention participant, containing information about AIDS, injecting drug users' risks for AIDS, drug treatment, general health facts, and social and health services available in the community.

Participants in the *enhanced* intervention received the same pre- and post-test counseling and educational brochures *with an additional four hours of group counseling* divided into three sessions. The enhanced intervention was designed to take participants through a sequence of attaining knowledge about HIV transmission, developing practical risk reduction skills (needle cleansing and condom use), empowering attitudinal and behavioral change, and developing a realistic plan to accomplish and maintain these changes (McCoy, Chitwood, Khoury, & Miles, 1990).

Outreach as a Mechanism for Behavioral Change

As can be seen from the results obtained from the Miami intervention program, both the standard and enhanced intervention participants were equally likely to indicate substantial levels of behavioral risk reduction. Focus groups of study participants were convened in an attempt to elicit the reasons for this lack of difference between the intervention groups. These individuals expressed the feeling that because of their contact with the outreach worker, they felt that someone cared about them and were looking out for them. Repeated street contact with the outreach worker, since he/she was a member of the project participants' neighborhood and/or culture, reinforced this feeling of caring and concern.

This ethnographic evidence indicated that the outreach worker can be as important an agent of change as the information and skills gained in the formal intervention program. The outreach worker has a high degree of credibility in the eyes of the target population, because he/she is a peer, a former drug user, and indigenous to the neighborhood from which study participants are recruited. His/her high visibility in the community introduces an element of continuity and a positive bonding relationship to an individual who, because of drug abuse, may feel socially isolated.

As the Miami site has received additional funding to continue its intervention in the Cooperative Agreement Risk Evaluation (CARE) Project, program principals have planned to increase the contact exposure of the indigenous outreach worker as a teacher and promoter of behavioral change among study participants. The outreach worker will stress risk reduction guidelines with project participants in informal street contact, thereby reinforcing the importance of the participant's continuing to reduce or eliminate AIDS-related risk behavior. More formal booster sessions will be provided to randomly-selected study participants at each follow-up session.

CONCLUSION

It is unusual, in the field of drug abuse prevention, to have followed a large cohort of non-institutionalized IDUs for such a long period of time. Administering a longitudinal design is expensive, requiring complicated, labor-intensive but necessary follow-up to establish the long-term effectiveness of a program.

While the Miami study had divided participants into standard and enhanced intervention groups, no practical difference was evident in their levels of risk reduction over 24 months of observations. Both groups exhibited equally substantial and sustained reductions in AIDS-related risk behavior. Such reductions were particularly evident in the area of drug use.

Intervention programs targeted to IDUs and their sexual partners must concentrate efforts within the neighborhoods where participants reside and/or frequent, identifying persons who can provide access to the group and credibility to the messages. Cultural knowledge and sensitivity to ethnic considerations are necessary elements of any risk reduction program. The use of indigenous outreach workers from the same racial/ethnic background as the target population was undoubtedly a major factor in the success of this program.

Effective intervention programs must also focus on both drug-using and sexual behavior and provide not only motivating information but also guide the development of specific technical and interpersonal skills that can provide the tangible means for changing high-risk behavior. Such programs must also be concerned with maintaining behavioral change once such change has been achieved.

The ultimate test of the effectiveness of risk reduction intervention programs concerns the extent to which positive behavior changes can be sustained over a long period of time. While fear can be a powerful short-term motivator of behavioral change, further analysis of data at longer term follow-up assessments provide the information to determine whether such dramatic reductions in AIDS-related risk behaviors have been retained over time.

The lessons learned from this demonstration project need to be refined and applied to the maintenance of behavior changes through long-term interventions ("booster sessions"), targeting subgroups for which the interventions were most successful. In addition, a determination should be made as to why elements of the interventions were not successful in other subgroups.

Public health, drug treatment, and other health care providers should be aware of successful outreach intervention strategies and incorporate them into state and local AIDS prevention programs targeting out-of-treatment drug users and their sexual partners. With increasing scarcity of public health funds, cost-efficiency must be as important a measure of success as program effectiveness.

The nation cannot afford to look to an overtaxed publicly-supported substance abuse treatment system to reduce HIV transmission cases arising from such risk behavior as needle sharing and unprotected sexual activity by IDUs–and definitely not as agencies for intervening with the sexual partners of IDUs. The prospects for expansion of treatment capacity, or changes in IDU attitudes toward acceptance of treatment, are not likely to change rapidly or dramatically. There is an urgent need to disseminate and implement effective and affordable intervention models of short duration (relative to traditional specialized treatment regimes or even the current demand-inspired attenuated ones) in order to reduce HIV transmission risks from these sources.

REFERENCES

Botvin, C. (1988). Defining "success" in drug abuse prevention. In *Problems of Drug Dependence, 1988: Proceedings of the 50th Annual Scientific Meeting.* Washington DC: US Government Printing Office.

Chitwood, D. D., Inciardi, J. A., McBride, D. C., McCoy, C. B., McCoy, H. V., & Trapido, E. (1991). *A Community approach to AIDS intervention: Exploring the Miami outreach project for injecting drug users and other high risk groups.* Westport, NC: Greenwood Press.

Clark, N. M. (1987). Social learning theory in current health education practice. In W. B. Ward, S. K. Simonds, P. D. Mullen, & M. H. Becker (Eds.), *Advances in health education and health education promotion, Vol. 2.* Greenwich, CN: JAI Press, Inc.

Coyle, S. L., Boruch, R. F., & Turner, C. F. (Eds.) (1991). *Evaluating AIDS prevention programs, expanded edition.* Washington, DC: National Academy of Science.

Des Jarlais, D. C., Friedman, S. R., & Hopkins, W. (1985). Risk reduction for the acquired immunodeficiency syndrome among intravenous drug users. *Annals of Internal Medicine, 313,* 755-759.

Donoghoe, M. C., Stimson, G. V., & Dolan, K. A. (1989). Sexual behavior of injecting drug users and associated risks of HIV infection for non-injecting sexual partners. *AIDS Care, 1,* 51-56.

Friedman, S. R., Des Jarlais, D. C., & Sotheran, J. (1986). AIDS health education for intravenous drug users. *Health Education Quarterly, 13,* 383-393.

Kroliczak, A., & Orange, L. (1992). First six NADR programs demonstrate effectiveness of community outreach. *Network, 2*(3), 1-7.

McCoy, C. B., Chitwood, D. D., Khoury, E. L., & Miles, C. E. (1990). The implementation of an experimental research design in the evaluation of an intervention to prevent AIDS among IV drug users. *The Journal of Drug Issues, 20*(2), 215-222.

McCoy, C. B., & Khoury, E. L. (1990). Drug use and the risk of AIDS. *American Behavioral Scientist, 33*(4), 419-431.

McCoy, C. B., & Khoury, E. L. (1992, April). *Community interventions for cancer and AIDS.* Paper presented at the Southern Sociological Society Annual Meetings, New Orleans, LA.

McCoy, C. B., Rivers, J. R., & Khoury, E. L. (1991, December). The role of epidemiologic and demographic data in substance abuse research and interventions. *Proceedings of the Community Epidemiology Work Group Meetings.* (pp. 475-482). Washington, DC: U.S. Government Printing Office.

McCoy, C. B., Weatherby, N. L., Miles, C. C., & Vogel, J. (1991). *Intervention services for high risk clients.* Report to the State of Florida Department of Health and Rehabilitative Services. Miami, FL: Comprehensive Drug Research Center.

Moss, A. R., & Chaisson, R. E. (1988). AIDS and Intravenous drug use in San Francisco. *AIDS and Public Policy Journal, 3*, 37-41.

Selwyn, P. A., Feiner, C., Cox, C. P., Lipshutz, C., & Cohen, R. L. (1987). Knowledge about AIDS and high-risk behavior among intravenous drug users in New York City. *AIDS, 1*, 247-254.

Snyder, F., Sowder, B., & Young, P. (1989). NIDA outreach demonstration projects provide insight into drug-use risk patterns. *Network, 1*(1), 1-7.

Strecher, V. J., Devellis, B. M., Becker, M. H., & Rosenstock, I. M. (1986). The role of self-efficacy in achieving health behavior change. *Health Education Quarterly, 13*, 359-371.

Turner, C. F., Miller, H. G., & Moses, L. E. (Eds.) (1989). Facilitating change in health behaviors. In *AIDS: Sexual behavior and intravenous drug use* (pp. 259-315). Washington, DC: National Academy Press.

Van Den Hoak, A. (1990, June). *Little change in sexual behavior in drug users in Amsterdam.* Presented at the Sixth International AIDS Conference, San Francisco, CA.

Watters, J. K. (1987). A street-based outreach model of AIDS prevention for intravenous drug users: Preliminary evaluation. *Contemporary Drug Problems, 14*, 411-423.

Weddington, W. W., Nemeth-Coslett, R., Anderson, M., Baxter, R., Baxter, S., Biernacki, P., Brown, B. S., McCoy, C. B. et al. (1990). Risk behaviors for HIV transmission amount intravenous-drug users not in treatment–United States, 1987-1989. *Morbidity and Mortality Weekly Report, 39*, 273-276.

Quantitative and Qualitative Methods to Assess Behavioral Change Among Injection Drug Users

Robert E. Booth, PhD
Stephen K. Koester, PhD
Charles S. Reichardt, PhD
J. Thomas Brewster, MSW

SUMMARY. The risk injecting drug users (IDUs) have for contracting the human immunodeficiency virus (HIV) led to governmental requests for interventions to prevent its spread. At the same time there was an urgent need to evaluate the effectiveness of these proposed interventions. We believe that both quantitative and qualita-

Robert E. Booth and Stephen K. Koester are affiliated with the Addiction Research and Treatment Services, Department of Psychiatry, University of Colorado School of Medicine. Charles S. Reichardt is associated with the Department of Psychology, University of Denver. J. Thomas Brewster is affiliated with the Addiction Research and Treatment Services, University of Colorado School of Medicine.

The authors wish to acknowledge the assistance of George Beschner and Barry Brown of the National Institute on Drug Abuse.

Please address correspondence and reprint requests to Robert Booth, Campus Box C-251, Department of Psychiatry, University of Colorado Health Sciences Center, 4200 East 9th Avenue, Denver, CO 80262.

Preparation of this article was supported by the National Institute on Drug Abuse, Contract No. 271-87-8208 and Grant DA-06912 and the National Institute on Alcohol Abuse and Alcoholism Grant U01-AA08778.

[Haworth co-indexing entry note]: "Quantitative and Qualitative Methods to Assess Behavioral Change Among Injection Drug Users." Booth, Robert E. et al. Co-published simultaneously in *Drugs & Society* (The Haworth Press, Inc.) Vol. 7, No. 3/4, 1993, pp. 161-183; and *AIDS and Community-Based Drug Intervention Programs: Evaluation and Outreach* (ed: Dennis G. Fisher, and Richard Needle) The Haworth Press, Inc., 1993, pp. 161-183. Multiple copies of this article/chapter may be purchased from The Haworth Document Delivery Center [1-800-3-HAWORTH; 9:00 a.m. - 5:00 p.m. (EST)].

Copyright © 1993 by Taylor & Francis

tive research methods should be employed in this effort. In this paper we discuss the differences between the two approaches, how they can complement one another, and present findings derived from their joint application to a particular risk behavior, needle sharing. Despite behavioral changes in a number of high risk activities, significant reductions in borrowing syringes were not reported by participants in structured interviews. Evidence obtained through participant observation and open-ended interviews indicated Colorado's paraphernalia law may have played a major role in encouraging this behavior.

Injection drug users (IDUs) are the second largest risk group in the United States for the human immunodeficiency virus (HIV). They are also the primary source for heterosexual transmission of the disease (CDC, 1990; Des Jarlais, & Friedman; Friedland, & Klein, 1987). HIV seropositivity is related to the frequency of drug injection, injection with used needles, sharing needles with others, injecting with strangers or acquaintances, injecting in shooting galleries, injection of cocaine, and injecting heroin and cocaine together (Chaisson et al. 1989; Chitwood et al. 1990; Des Jarlais et al., 1989; Page, Chitwood, Smith, Kane, & McBride, 1990; Schoenbaum et al., 1989; Wiebel, 1988).

For women, injection drug use is the single greatest HIV risk factor, followed by sexual relations with an IDU (Guinan, & Hardy, 1987). More than half of non-injecting women infected with HIV through heterosexual intercourse have been infected through a male IDU (Cohen, Haver, & Wofsey, 1989). Drug injecting female prostitutes have more than three times the infection rate of prostitutes who are not IDUs (CDC, 1987).

Beginning in 1986, the Centers for Disease Control (CDC) requested applications for projects designed to modify the behaviors that placed drug injectors at risk for HIV. The following year, the National Institute on Drug Abuse (NIDA) also requested applications for demonstration projects to address the rising epidemic. The intervention from which the present work emerged was a response to the NIDA initiative. To assess the efficacy of the intervention with IDUs, both qualitative and quantitative research methods were employed. The present paper focuses on the strengths of using both of these approaches. Together the two methods offer the opportunity to achieve a greater understanding than could be attained with either method alone. An illustration of the joint application of the methods will be presented, along with some of the policy implications derived from their results.

QUANTITATIVE AND QUALITATIVE RESEARCH APPROACHES

A distinction is often drawn between quantitative and qualitative research (Guba, 1978; Patton, 1978). The next few paragraphs describe some of the distinguishing features of these two types of research approaches.

Quantitative researchers typically study large samples of subjects through experimental, quasi-experimental, or survey research designs. Researchers test hypotheses using structured questionnaires and multivariate inferential statistical techniques. From experimental studies in the laboratory, where extraneous elements are regulated, to evaluating program effectiveness, where contaminating variables are accounted for through design and measurement, quantitative methods are utilized to gain systematic knowledge with emphasis on the replicability of results. Quantitative research emphasizes objectivity and is oriented toward verification, with generalizations to other populations who have not been tested (Reichardt, & Cook, 1979).

Random assignment of subjects and double blind strategies for measurement are often considered hallmarks of experimental design. Where such methods are not feasible, as in many applied research settings, quasi-experimental designs are employed as the next best alternative. Because all measures have some degree of error, and are thus approximations of "truth," statistical methods are needed to assess "probabilities" and create "confidence intervals."

In contrast, qualitative researchers study relatively small numbers of subjects, using participant observation, open-ended interviewing techniques, focus groups, and ethnography. Researchers who employ these methods, typically sociologists or anthropologists, attempt to explain the way of life or behavior of a culture from the perspective of group members. Methods tend to be naturalistic, inductive, and holistic (Guba, 1978; Patton, 1978; Reichardt, &

Cook, 1979). Qualitative research is often employed for the purpose of discovery or hypothesis generation. To accomplish this, qualitative research emphasizes research methods that promote interaction between the researcher and the subjects. Observation and interviewing techniques that allow subjects to speak in their own voice are the tools used to achieve this degree of understanding.

The most comprehensive form of qualitative research is ethnography, which seeks to produce an in-depth, descriptive study of a group or culture. Traditionally, ethnographers produce this detailed, case study of a group of people by living and working among them for a prolonged period. Today, researchers also employ ethnographic methods in studies where this degree of immersion is impractical or unnecessary. This intensive approach is meant to lend to an "emic" or insider perspective of the subject group. Methods commonly used by ethnographers include the collection of archival data, census information, life histories, and household surveys. Two complimentary qualitative research methods are also integral to all ethnographic studies: participant observation and open-ended interviewing techniques.

Participant observation involves interacting with subjects in their own environment and on their own terms. It enables the researcher to understand the context in which people live, and it allows the researcher to compare what people say with what they actually do. Understanding the physical and social setting of people's lives, as well as the social, political, and economic forces affecting them is essential for explaining their actions. Actually witnessing people engage in the behavior being studied contributes to its understanding and provides key details that might be overlooked in self-report data. In an earlier study, for example, participant observation enabled us to see the multiple ways in which HIV can be transmitted during the preparation of drugs for injection (Koester, Booth, & Wiebel, 1990).

Qualitative interviewing techniques range from informal conversations to semi-structured, directed attempts to gain specific information. Focused, open-ended interviews can provide answers to a particular question or serve to explain an observed behavior pattern. More informal conversations can be equally revealing, allowing the subject to determine what information is important, often leading the researcher into areas of inquiry that would otherwise have been missed. These interview techniques are well suited for gathering information regarded as sensitive and unlikely to be uncovered in more formal structured interviews (Herdt, & Boxer, 1992; Trotter, 1992).

Focus groups are another open-ended interviewing technique that, until recently, have principally been used as a marketing tool rather than as a research method. Although this technique often takes place in an unnatural and controlled setting, it can prove to be useful because it enables the researcher to gain a large amount of information in a relatively short period of time. In focus groups the researcher facilitates the group in a discussion (Morgan, 1988). In our research, this interview method has been used to inform questionnaire development and intervention design.

Quantitative and qualitative methods each have their own strengths and weaknesses. Qualitative methods, by employing unstructured or semistructured methods, do not force the subject to address the preconceived theories of the researcher. Respondents are offered the opportunity to describe their feelings and observations in an unobtrusive manner. One of the advantages of qualitative methods is their sensitivity to the subtle nuances in the thoughts and interpretations of those studied. Another advantage is the ability to quickly change the line of questioning as unanticipated discoveries occur. Open-ended answers often allow the respondent to communicate more elusive ideas than close-ended answers. Participation observation permits group members to behave as they normally would, without intrusion.

On the other hand, the lack of structure, combined with, generally, small samples, opens qualitative methodologies to attacks of lacking in representativeness and the charge of subjectivity. Human perception is susceptible to bias. Over-involvement with members of the culture being studied, sometimes referred to as "going native," threatens the scientific objectivity of researchers when they abandon their analytical perspective by uncritically accepting the views of the members (Adler, & Adler, 1987; Gold, 1958; Hammersley, & Atkinson, 1983).

Quantitative methods were devised as a means to avoid or reduce some of these biases. The use of large samples by quantitative researchers allows for small effects to be detected and increases the generalizability of results. Studies can be replicated at different times and by different researchers, creating a body of scientific knowledge on particular subjects of interest, such as evidenced by the vast literature on conditioning theory. These advantages are often achieved, however, at some loss of a depth of understanding that qualitative knowing is adept at providing. In addition, the use of formal interviews and structured questionnaires introduces a foreign element into the social setting and is open to biases in the interpretation of both the format and content of the questions by the subject (Katz, 1942; Cantril, 1944; Webb et al., 1966). Even the act of measuring itself presents the potential for reactions to what is being tested (Campbell, & Stanley, 1966; Webb, Campbell, Schwartz, Sechrest 1966).

Although some have argued that because the two methods are founded upon disparate philosophical foundations the two methods themselves are incompatible (Guba, 1978), it would appear obvious that much could be gained by combining the two methodological approaches. This is because the strengths of one method can often be used to counterbalance the weaknesses of the other. The depth achieved through qualitative research, for example, could aid in the interpretation of inconsistent or confusing quantitative findings. Similarly, the nature of the relationship between behaviors, or the question of how widespread a particular observed behavior is, could be assessed through the use of quantitative methods (Trend, 1978).

With the appearance of the Acquired Immune Deficiency Syndrome (AIDS), and the response of federal, state and local agencies requesting proposals to prevent the further spread of the disease, there was an urgent need to develop interventions that were relevant to the needs of high risk groups and to assess their viability. We believe that both qualitative and quantitative research methods of inquiry should be brought to bear on the issue. Though the use of these approaches in combination has been proposed before (Britan, 1978; Campbell, 1974; Reichardt, & Cook, 1979; Trow, 1957) they have been implemented in practice with surprising infrequency (Denzin, 1970; Garner, 1954; Webb et al., 1966).

Because the present paper is intended, primarily, to illustrate what can be learned about risk for HIV by using qualitative and quantitative methods together, rather than to be a methodological tutorial, specific details on methodology will be brief. Similarly, qualitative observations on the neighborhoods and drug use patterns that are not central to the current discussion will be limited. More thorough examinations of these issues are available elsewhere (Booth, Booth, Koester, Brewster, Wiebel, & Fritz, 1991; Booth, & Wiebel, in press; Booth, & Watters, in press; Koester, 1988; Koester, in press).

METHODS:
EVALUATING NEEDLE-RELATED RISK REDUCTION

Quantitative

Beginning in 1989 a quantitative assessment was undertaken to assess the effectiveness of a street-based intervention in modifying HIV risk behaviors related to the use of needles. The population of interest consisted of drug injectors not in treatment, recruited from targeted, social networks through multiple snowball sampling (Goodman, 1961). Individuals from the neighborhoods selected for intervention, who were also familiar with the drug subculture, were hired to serve as outreach staff. Their role as prevention workers included establishing rapport within IDU networks and encouraging members to adopt safer needle and sexual practices. As primary contacts with IDUs they also functioned as research assistants, recruiting subjects for structured interviews. To be interviewed, respondents had to be at least 18 years of age, not currently enrolled in treatment, and to have injected drugs within the previous six months, according to self-report verified through examination for scarred tissue. Interviewers were professionally trained and, like the outreach workers, former participants in the drug subculture.

Respondents were interviewed at two points in time using structured questionnaires (AIDS Initial Assessment, versions 6 and 8, and AIDS Follow-up Assessment, version 1) exploring various needle risk activities during the six months preceding the interview. These included the frequency of injection, renting and borrowing needles, sharing cookers, injecting at a shooting gallery, and use of disinfectants such as bleach. In addition, data on overall drug injection in the 30 days prior to the interview were collected. The interview schedules and protocols were approved by the Human Subjects Committee and all subjects were compensated for their participation.

To aid in the interpretation of findings, change in risk behaviors was assessed using the Wilcoxon signed-ranks test for matched pairs, a procedure that incorporates the magnitude of differences. In addition to the analysis of individual risk behaviors, a composite-dichotomous risk index was created based on the variables measuring injecting, injecting in a shooting gallery, renting or borrowing needles, sharing a cooker, and use of bleach, alcohol, or boiling water to disinfect needles. Subjects in the low risk category either: (a) did not inject in the six months prior to their interview; or, (b) they injected but not in a shooting gallery and did not rent or borrow needles nor did they share a cooker; or, (c) they participated in at least one of these behaviors but reported using disinfectants 100% of the time. High risk respondents engaged in one or more of these risk behaviors but did not always use a disinfectant. For this analysis, the chi-square test for differences in proportions was utilized with the Yates correction.

Qualitative

Outreach workers, acting as key informants, introduced the project's anthropologist to groups of active IDUs in the targeted neighborhoods. Participant observation of these neighborhoods' drug scenes and the drug-using behavior within them was combined with open-ended interviews with local drug injectors to gain an understanding of high-risk drug behavior. This ethnographic fieldwork, conducted at the same time as the collection of quantitative data, took place in a well known, highly visible drug copping location on Denver's eastside. General topics discussed with injectors included personal histories, drug-using behavior, daily routines, and knowledge of HIV. Through these open-ended interviews the anthropologist established a level of acceptance that resulted in informal but increasingly intimate conversations. With this acceptance, it was possible to extend observational research into the neighborhood's copping areas, bars, apartments, parks and shooting galleries, and observe users buying drugs and preparing them for injection.

Through the serendipity that often occurs in conjunction with participant observation, the content of the fieldwork took on an interesting addition. In the process of observing drug copping activities, the anthropologist was stopped, searched by the police, and asked what he was doing in the area. This experience was observed by everyone on the street and served to reduce suspicion toward the researcher. It also led to a more detailed examination of the effect of law enforcement on risk behavior.

In a series of open-ended interviews on this topic, injectors discussed how police activity affected the way they used drugs. These interviews revealed a pattern, and led to the hypothesis that various aspects of law enforcement encouraged street-based drug users to share a common syringe. Continued discussions with users about police activities followed, along with a survey administered to 24 neighborhood injectors. A convenience sample of injectors, recruited by outreach workers, were asked a set of questions by the workers and their answers recorded. Questions included: Did they carry a syringe and, if not, why? Had they ever been cited for possession of a syringe? How did they obtain syringes? This survey was followed by semi-structured, open-ended interviews with injectors in another high profile drug neighborhood in Denver, and brief discussions with police officers about their enforcement activities. Some interviews were tape recorded in the project office. Additional discussions, observations and open-ended interviews took place in the neighborhoods and were recorded as field notes.

RESULTS: NEEDLE-RELATED RISK REDUCTION

Quantitative

The 178 subjects included in the quantitative assessment of needle-related risk factors averaged 34.6 years of age (SD = 7.59, range 18-59), with 57% between the ages of 30 and 40. Men accounted for 65% of the sample. In terms of ethnic composition, 55% were Black, 26% Hispanic and 17% White. In the six months prior to the interview, 34% of the respondents reported their major source of income was a legitimate job, while 39% reported their primary source was from illegal activities. Overall, 58% of the respondents had received illegal income during this time period. At the time of their initial interview, 62% were unemployed, 10% worked full-time, and 8% part-time.

The average time between interviews was 8.7 months (SD = 3.5). Although a follow-up rate of only 41% was achieved (178/435), this figure is not an accurate reflection of follow-up efforts. When the project began recruiting subjects, respondents were told by interviewers that they could fabricate a date of birth. This was done to gain their trust by insuring anonymity. During the first wave of follow-up interviews the error of this decision became obvious: It was virtually impossible to match interview schedules, because names were not recorded and respondents rarely recalled the birth date they had made-up earlier. As a result, individuals presenting themselves for the second interview were turned away when their subject number could not be determined. In actuality, 68% presented themselves for their follow-up interview.

To test whether those interviewed at time two were representative of the total cohort, respondents at time two were compared with those lost to follow-up using data from the initial interview. Ethnically, Blacks had the lowest drop-out rate and Anglos the highest (51% and 75%, respectively, $p < .01$). No significant difference was found on the frequency of injection, however one significant effect was observed relative to HIV risk: Those not re-interviewed reported more needle borrowing than those who were re-interviewed (68% and 56%, respectively, $p < .01$).

All respondents reported IV drug use during the six months prior to their initial interview. Overall, 89% had injected cocaine, 71% heroin and 56% speedballs, which is the combination of heroin and cocaine injected together. Drugs most frequently injected on a daily basis at baseline were heroin (33%), cocaine (26%) and speedballs (18%). In terms of risk behaviors related to the use of needles, 39% reported they had rented and 66% borrowed needles during the six months before the first interview, 85% had shared a cooker, and 38% had injected in a shooting gallery, a location where needle renting is common. Use of bleach to disinfect needles was indicated by 42%, including 6% who did so every time they injected.

Statistically significant changes in the frequency of injection following the intervention was observed on each of the three drugs most commonly used in the six months before the interview and in the overall frequency of drug injection in the previous 30 days (Figure 1). Daily injection of cocaine declined from 26% of the study participants to 9%, heroin from 33% to 16%, speedballs from 18% to 6%, and overall frequency of drug injection from 40% to 21%.

In the pre-post analysis with the composite index (Figure 2), significant reductions in risk behaviors were observed across time ($Z = \$3.80, p < .000$). Of the 145 high risk subjects at the time of the initial interview, 31% were low risk at follow-up, reducing the percentage of high risk subjects from 84% to 65%.

Figure 3 illustrates change in needle related risks. As these data show, significant change occurred in renting needles and frequenting shooting galleries. Although not shown, positive change was also noted in the use of bleach ($Z = \$2.82, p < .02$. However, a lack of significant change was observed in borrowing needles, perhaps the principle behavior outreach workers sought to impact, and sharing cookers.

Qualitative

Qualitative research findings suggest that there was little change in the "borrowing" or exchange of used needles between street-based drug injectors largely because syringes were usually in scarce supply when they were ready to inject. Many users refused to carry syringes, a consequence of both a Colorado state statute and a Denver municipal ordinance (Koester, 1989; Koester, 1991). These laws define hypodermic syringes as drug paraphernalia if their intended use is "to introduce into the human body any controlled substance under circumstances in violation of the laws of the state" (CRS 12-22-501). The penalty for this misdemeanor offense is a maximum $100 fine (Figure 4).

These laws are based on a model written in 1979 by the Drug Enforcement Agency (DEA) as a way to regulate the sale and possession of drug paraphernalia. The purpose was to establish a standardized definition that could be adopted by states and municipalities (Pascal, 1988). Currently, 48 states and the District of Columbia have laws regulating paraphernalia based upon this DEA model. In addition, 12 states require a prescription to purchase a syringe (Fernando, 1991). Restricting paraphernalia is viewed as a

Figure 1. Change In Daily Drug Injection

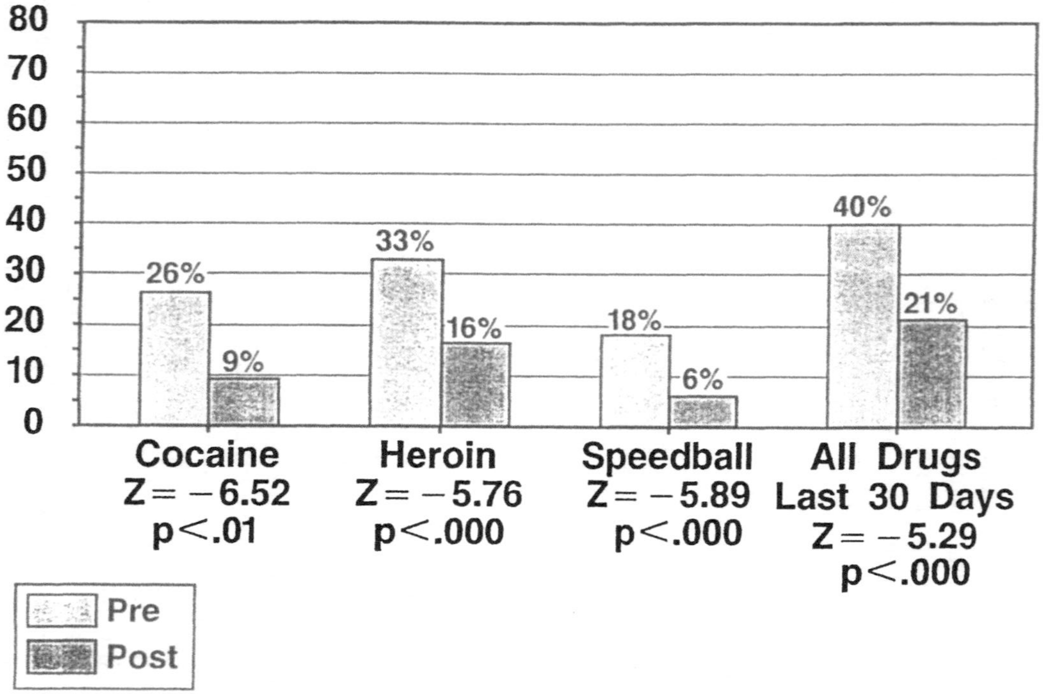

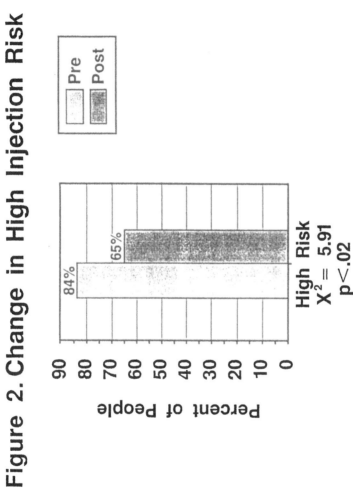

Figure 2. Change in High Injection Risk

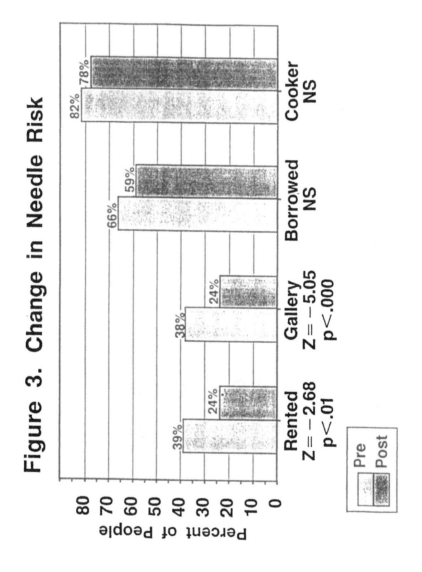

Figure 3. Change in Needle Risk

Figure 4.

COLORADO REVISED STATUTE

12-22-501 CONTROL OF DRUG PARAPHERNALIA

The general assembly hereby finds and declares that the
possession, sale, manufacture, delivery, or advertisement of
drug paraphernalia results in the legitimization and
encouragement of the illegal use of controlled substances by
making the drug culture more visible and enticing and that the
ready availability of drug paraphernalia tends to promote,
suggest, or increase the public acceptability of the illegal use of
controlled substances.

way to restrain drug abuse and provide law enforcement with an additional tool to fight it. In the case of syringes this approach has been effective; because their possession is a crime, they are a scarce commodity on the street. Unfortunately, this has also acted to encourage borrowing needles. As Feldman and Biernacki (1988) note:

> The illegality of possessing hypodermic syringes . . . accounts for the unpredictable supply of hypodermic syringes, the chronic fear of arrest, and the necessity of constructing social arrangements that involve needle sharing. (p. 35)

This same sequence of events has been observed in the highly visible, eastside drug copping areas in Denver where we conducted our research and was confirmed by the street-based users that frequent it. Drug injectors in this community rarely carry syringes. As one user explained:

> One thing you will not catch is someone (on the eastside) just walking around carrying a needle. You'll catch them with dope before you'll catch them with a needle.

This injector's reaction was substantiated through on-going field-work, discussions with neighborhood drug injectors, and a survey of 24 injectors, 23 of whom stated that they did not carry syringes because they were afraid of arrest.

At first, this reaction to a petty offense seems ludicrous when, in the course of a single day, these same injectors may commit far more serious offenses, including buying and using illicit drugs and engaging in illegal activities to obtain them. However, for poor, street-based drug users these crimes are unavoidable. Attempts are made to minimize their risk by controlling the times and places they commit them. It is not as easy to limit the period in which one carries a syringe. Often, there is a significant time lag between purchasing a syringe and obtaining the drug. During this period the individual is vulnerable to arrest. Unlike crimes committed because the user is addicted and supporting a habit, this offense can be avoided. As a local injector explained:

> Addicts don't normally worry about getting a fit until after they cop their dope. Nobody wants to put a fit in their pocket until after they get their dope. Only time you'll see somebody hanging around is when they're trying to speedball. They may already have their heroin and they're waiting for the cocaine man to come through.

Injectors in this neighborhood are particularly susceptible to the enforcement of the paraphernalia law because of the high profile they must maintain, due in part to an impoverished lifestyle that results in temporary living arrangements. This visibility is especially pronounced when they are engaged in drug copping and support their habit by "running" or touting drugs for local dealers. This particular hustle requires the runner to actively seek out buyers, take their money to the dealer, and return with the drug. In exchange for assuming the high degree of risk accompanying this conspicuous behavior, the runner is given a "taste" or small amount of the drug by the buyer. The risk of supporting a habit by running, and thus carrying drugs, is further accentuated by the almost constant presence of the police. Carrying a syringe under such circumstances compounds the chance of arrest.

These street-based users are more likely to have drugs on them, which are easier to hide, than a syringe. Police will almost certainly find a syringe when conducting a search but are far less likely to find drugs, largely because users can rarely afford to purchase more than a small quantity at a time and drugs can be carried in one's mouth. If stopped, the police may not detect the drug and, if suspected, it can be quickly swallowed.

If an injector is caught with a syringe he is normally issued a citation requiring a court appearance. If the user pleads guilty or no contest, he receives a fine of $50 to $100. A user can, of course, plead not guilty and have a trial. None of the users surveyed for this investigation, or who were talked to during the course of two years of fieldwork, knew of anyone who pled not guilty. While the threat of the fine is enough to discourage possessing a syringe, the actual consequence of an arrest is often far more serious. This is because street-based users often fail to appear in court for misdemeanor charges and, as a result, have outstanding bench warrants. When stopped by police, an identification check will reveal these warrants and the individual will go to jail. Feldman and Biernacki (1988) report a similar conclusion:

> The illegality of hypodermic syringes prevents many publicly labeled addicts from keeping needles in their possession, since another arrest for 'old times' may result in jail sentences. For those persons with previous incarcerations, the periods in jail have been bitter experiences which they dread and strive to avoid repeating. (p. 35)

The lack of significant change among respondents in regard to sharing cookers is consistent with the finding showing little change in borrowing needles. Repeated participant observation with users preparing drugs for injection shows how these activities occur together. This is particularly the case when users have combined their money to purchase a drug. When street-based injectors share the cost of a drug, they almost always divide it by mixing it first in a single container or cooker. The drug is then divided by using the calibrations on the barrel of the syringe. The first user will draw up the entire liquified solution into the syringe and then either squirt the other person's share back into the cooker, or simply inject his share, leaving the other person's in the just-used syringe. Sharing the cost of drugs and users' desire to prepare drugs as quickly as possible encourage the sharing of cookers, even when each user has their own syringe (Koester, Booth, & Wiebel, 1990).

Another explanation for the lack of change in this risk activity is that outreach prevention efforts did not address this behavior until relatively late in the project. In fact, through ethnographic fieldwork in shooting galleries it was observed that IDUs shared a number of items, other than needles, in the process of injecting, including water, cotton, and cookers (Koester, Booth, & Wiebel, 1990). Knowledge of these risk behaviors led to changes in the message outreach workers imparted to those with whom they intervened.

DISCUSSION

Our observation that a Colorado state statute and Denver city ordinance regulating syringe possession may actually serve to encourage needle sharing among drug injectors was based upon findings from a combined qualitative and quantitative research effort. Data from NIDA's structured questionnaire showed that, although drug injectors in Denver had made significant strides in changing some high risk behaviors, little change was seen in regard to borrowing previously used syringes. At the same time, independently collected research findings from a qualitative assessment, performed in the same neighborhoods where subjects were recruited for formal interviews, revealed that street-based injectors rarely carried needles, even when engaged in buying drugs for their own consumption. Injectors explained this seemingly inconsistent behavior as a response to these laws and their penalties. As a result, IDUs frequently found themselves in situations where they used whatever syringe was available. To further test the validity of this finding, we have incorporated a series of supplemental questions to NIDA's current structured questionnaire, the Risk Behavior Assessment. These questions are based on information provided by our qualitative research. By adding them to our quantitative instrument we will be able to verify our results with a sample larger than available through conventional qualitative methods.

Qualitative methods were also employed in the development of structured interview questions for our studies of drug injectors.

Without knowing the context within which various behaviors occur, questions thought to be addressing needle sharing, for example, were likely to be misinterpreted. IDUs who inject and share a syringe purchased together typically respond negatively to questions about how often they use someone else's syringe (e.g., "In the last 30 days when you used drugs with a needle, how many times did you use works that someone *lent* and gave you that you know had been used by someone else?"). On the other hand, asking how often an injector shared a syringe implies a degree of intimacy that if, non-existent, will illicit a negative response. By understanding the context of injecting behavior, questions can be constructed that subjects understand in the *way* in which quantitative researchers intend (e.g., "How many times in the last 30 days did you inject using works that you know had been *used* by someone else?").

We have also utilized quantitative and qualitative methods in the assessment of our "delivery system" (Rossi, 1978). Outreach staff serve as interventionists in helping reduce risks associated with HIV. Their work on the streets is, for the most part, unstructured and dynamic. This raises a number of questions, such as: Are the interventions being delivered as planned? Are subjects recruited according to the sampling procedures? What differences are there between individual outreach workers? To answer these questions we employ both of the approaches described in this paper. Subjects are interviewed, using a structured questionnaire, about their contacts with outreach staff from our project and others, the nature of those contacts, how often they received prevention materials, how often they were referred for medical or drug treatment, and their overall impression of outreach efforts. Through participation observation we are also able to view outreach efforts first hand. In addition, semi-structured open-ended interviews with project participants provide further information about the delivery system.

CONCLUSION

AIDS is a behaviorally transmitted disease presently without a vaccine or cure. The only means of preventing its spread is to change the behaviors responsible for it. Since the mid 1980s, both federally-funded programs and community-based efforts have made dramatic progress in educating members of high risk populations about ways to modify their behavior, and thus reduce the risk of infection. Social and behavioral scientists have played a key role informing these interventions and evaluating their success. Far less has been accomplished, however, in changing the environmental conditions which serve to promote high risk behavior. As shown by our illustration, such conditions may compromise efforts based on cognitive models emphasizing individual behavior change.

Combining quantitative and qualitative research methodologies to study why drug injectors share needles has led us to conclude that laws regulating the possession of syringes have become counterproductive. Paraphernalia laws were written in response to this nation's drug abuse, before HIV had become a recognized epidemic. Today, HIV is arguably an even greater health crisis than drug abuse. Integrating quantitative and qualitative research methods has enabled us to understand how this law encourages risky behavior. If the intent of the law is "To protect and promote the public peace, health, safety and welfare . . . " (CRS 12-22-501) then our research suggests it should be amended to exclude syringes. Without the fear of arrest, we may find greater compliance with intervention messages urging IDUs not to inject with used needles of others.

REFERENCES

Adler, P. A., & Adler, P. (1987). *Membership roles in field research.* Newbury Park: Sage.

Booth, R. E., Koester, S., Brewster, J. T., Wiebel, W. W., & Fritz, R. (1991). Intravenous drug users and AIDS: Risk behaviors. *The American Journal on Drug and Alcohol Abuse. 17,* 337-353.

Booth, R. E., Wiebel, W. W. (in press). The effectiveness of reducing needle related risks for HIV through indigenous outreach to injection drug users. *The American Journal on Addictions.*

Booth, R. E., Watters, J. K. (in press). A factor analytic approach to modeling AIDS risk behaviors among heterosexual injection drug users. *Journal of Drug Issues.*

Britan, G. M. (1978). Experimental and contextual models of program evaluation. *Evaluation and Program Planning, 1,* 229-234.

Campbell, D. T. (1974, September). *Qualitative knowing in action research.* Paper presented at 82nd annual meeting of the American Psychological Association, New Orleans, LA.

Campbell, D. T., and Stanley, J. C. (1966). *Experimental and quasi-experimental design for research.* Chicago: Rand McNally.

Cantril, H. (1944). *Gaging public opinion.* New Jersey: Princeton University Press.

CDC [Centers for Disease Control]. (1987). *Human immunodeficiency virus infection in the United States: a review of current knowledge, 36,* 1-48.

CDC [Center for Disease Control]. (1990, February). *HIV Monthly Surveillance Report.*

Chaisson, R. E., Bacchetti, P., Osmond, D., Brodie, B., Sande, M. A., & Moss, A. R. (1989). Cocaine use and HIV infection in intravenous drug users in San Francisco. *Journal of the American Medical Association, 261,* 561-565.

Chitwood, D. D., McCoy, B., Inciardi, J. A., McBride, D. C., Comerford, M., Trapido, E., McCoy, V., Page, J. B., Griffin, J., Fletcher, M. A., & Ashman, M. S. (1990). HIV Seropositivity of needles from shooting galleries in south Florida. *American Journal of Public Health, 80,* 150-152.

Cohen, J. B., Haver, L. B., Wofsey, C. B. (1989). Women and intravenous drugs: Parenteral and heterosexual transmission of human immunodeficiency virus. *Journal of Drug Issues, 19,* 39-56.

Denzin, N. (1970). *The Research act.* Chicago: Aldine.

Des Jarlais, D. C., Friedman, S. R. (1987). HIV infection among intravenous drug users: Epidemiology and risk reduction. *AIDS, 1,* 67-76.

Des Jarlais, D. C., Friedman, S. R., Novick, D. M., Sotheran, J. L., Thomas, P., Yancovitz, S. R., Mildvan, D., Weber, J., Kreek, M. J., Maslansky, R., Bartelme, S., Spira, T., & Marmor, M. (1989). HIV-1 infection among intravenous drug users in Manhattan, New York City, from 1977 through 1987. *Journal of the American Medical Association, 261,* 1008-1012.

Feldman, H., & Biernacki, P. (1988). The ethnography of needle sharing among intravenous drug users and implications for public policies and intervention strategies. In R. J. Battjes & R. W. Pickens (Eds.), National and International perspectives, *Needle Sharing Among Intravenous Drug Users:* Washington DC: National Institute on Drug Abuse, Monograph 80.

Fernando, D. (1991). Commentary: Fundamental limitations of needle exchange programs as a strategy for HIV prevention among IVDUs in the US. *AIDS and Public Policy, 6,* 113-120.

Friedland, G. H., Klein, R. S. (1987). Transmission of the human immunodeficiency virus. *New England Journal of Medicine, 317,* 1125-1135.

Garner, W. R. (1954). Context effects and the validity of a loudness scale. *Journal of Experimental Psychology, 48,* 218-224.

Gold, R. L. (1958). Roles in sociological field observation. *Social Forces, 36,* 217-223.

Goodman, L. A. (1961). Snowball sampling. *Annuals of Mathematical Statistics, 32,* 148-170.

Guba, E. (1978). Toward a methodology of naturalistic inquiry in educational evaluation. *CSE Monograph Series in Evaluation.* Los Angeles: Center for the Study of Evaluation, UCLA Graduate School of Education.

Guinan, M. E., & Hardy, A. (1987). Epidemiology of AIDS in women in the United States, 1981 through 1986. *Journal of the American Medical Association, 257*, 19-22.

Hammersley, M., & Atkinson, P. (1983). *Ethnography: Principles in practice.* New York: Tavistock.

Herdt, G., & Boxer, A. M. (1992). *Ethnographic issues in the study of AIDS.* Manuscript in preparation.

Katz, D. (1942). Do interviews bias poll results? *Public Opinion Quarterly, 6*, 248-268.

Koester, S. (1988, October). *Ethnography and AIDS: A view from Denver.* Paper presented at the First International Symposium on Education and Information about AI DS, Ixtapa, MX.

Koester, S. (1989, April). *When push comes to shove: Poverty, law enforcement and high risk activity.* Paper presented at the Annual Meeting of the Society for Applied Anthropology, Santa Fe, NM.

Koester, S. (February, 1991). Why do they share: Ethnography and needle sharing. Paper presented at the Annual Meeting of the American Association for the Advancement of Science, Washington, D.C.

Koester, S. (in press). Applying an outreach-oriented public health model in three Denver neighborhoods. *Community based research and AIDS.*

Koester, S. K., Booth, R. E., & Wiebel, W. W. (1990). The risk of HIV transmission from sharing water, drug-mixing containers and cotton filters among intravenous drug users. *The International Journal of Drug Policy, 1*, 28-30.

Morgan, D. L. (1988). Focus groups as qualitative research. *Qualitative Research Methods Series, 16*, Newbury Park: Sage.

Page, B. J., Chitwood, D. D., Smith, P. C., Kane, N., & McBride, D. C. (1990). Intravenous drug use and HIV infection in Miami. *Medical Anthropology Quarterly, 4*, 56-71.

Pascal, C. (1988). Intravenous drug abuse and AIDS transmission: Federal and state laws regulating needle availability. In R. J. Battjes & R. W. Pickens (eds.), National and International Perspectives. *Needle sharing among intravenous drug users:* Washington D.C.: National Institute on Drug Abuse, Monograph 80.

Patton, M. Q. (1978). *Utilization-focused evaluation.* Newbury Park, CA: Sage.

Reichardt, C. S., & Cook, T. D. (1979). Beyond qualitative versus quantitative methods. *Qualitative and Quantitative Methods in Evaluation Research.* 7-32.

Rossi, P. H. (1978). Issues in the evaluation of human services delivery. *Evaluation Quarterly, 2*, 573-599.

Schoenbaum, E. E., Hartel, D., Selwyn, P. A., Klein, R. S., Davenny, K., Rogers, M., Feiner, C., & Friedland, G. (1989). Risk factors for human immunodeficiency virus infection in intravenous drug users. *New England Journal of Medicine, 321*, 874-879.

Trend, M. G. (1978). On the reconciliation of qualitative and quantitative analyses, A case study. *Human Organization, 37*, 345-354.

Trotter, R. T. (1992). *Preparation for fieldwork: Lessons from ethnographic field-work.* Manuscript in preparation.

Trow, M. (1957). Comment on participant observation and interviewing: A comparison. *Human Organization, 16,* 33-35.

Webb, E. J., Campbell, D. T., Schwartz, R. D., & Sechrest, L. (1966). *Unobtrusive measures: nonreactive research in the social sciences.* Chicago: Rand McNally.

Wiebel, W. (1988). Study of IV drug users and AIDS finds differing infection rate, risk behaviors. [Letter to the editor] *Journal of the American Medical Association, 260,* 3105.

Using Goal-Oriented Counseling and Peer Support to Reduce HIV/AIDS Risk Among Drug Users Not in Treatment

Fen Rhodes, PhD
Gary L. Humfleet, PhD

SUMMARY. A six-month HIV/AIDS risk intervention program for injection drug and crack users not in treatment is described, incorporating behavioral contracting, social support, and social modeling as core elements. The program utilizes goal-oriented behavioral counseling and HIV testing in conjunction with social support by peers and project outreach workers to facilitate personal change by drug-using participants. The intervention incorporates both group workshops and individual counseling sessions plus monthly social events for participants, supportive peers, and project staff. Local drug users who have successfully reduced their own risk of HIV/AIDS are utilized as positive role models for risk reduction. In addition, outreach workers maintain structured supportive contacts with program par-

Fen Rhodes and Gary L. Humfleet are affiliated with the AIDS Research & Education Project, Department of Psychology, California State University, Long Beach, Long Beach, CA 90840.

This research is supported by a grant from the National Institute on Drug Abuse (U01-DA07474).

[Haworth co-indexing entry note]: "Using Goal-Oriented Counseling and Peer Support to Reduce HIV/AIDS Risk Among Drug Users Not in Treatment." Rhodes, Fen, and Gary L. Humfleet. Co-published simultaneously in *Drugs & Society* (The Haworth Press, Inc.) Vol. 7, No. 3/4, 1993, pp. 185-204; and: *AIDS and Community-Based Drug Intervention Programs: Evaluation and Outreach* (ed: Dennis G. Fisher, and Richard Needle) The Haworth Press, Inc., 1993, pp. 185-204. Multiple copies of this article/chapter may be purchased from The Haworth Document Delivery Center [1-800-3-HAWORTH; 9:00 a.m. - 5:00 p.m. (EST)].

Copyright © 1993 by Taylor & Francis

ticipants on a scheduled basis. The efficacy of this enhanced intervention program in comparison with standard HIV testing and AIDS education is currently being evaluated in a follow-up study.

It has been demonstrated that drug users, in particular those injecting drugs, who participate in Human Immunodeficiency Virus (HIV) educational interventions outside of drug treatment programs can and do modify their behavior to reduce personal risk of HIV infection (Bruneau et al., 1991; Chitwood et al., 1990; Iguchi, Watters, & Biernacki, 1990; Liebman, McIlvaine et al., 1990; Moss & Chaisson, 1988; National AIDS Research Consortium, 1990; Neaigus et al., 1990; Tross et al., 1991). Such interventions frequently provide HIV transmission and prevention information in the context of informal interactions between outreach workers and drug users on the street (e.g., Chitwood et al., 1990; Neaigus et al., 1990). Formal risk education and counseling sessions in group or individual formats, as a rule incorporating both cognitive and motivational components, may also be held in storefronts or other neighborhood facilities (e.g., Liebman, Bowden et al., 1990). The number of formal sessions may vary, but typically this number ranges between two and four. The distribution of bleach and condoms by outreach workers and counselors has come to be an integral part of HIV intervention programs for out-of-treatment drug users (Moss & Chaisson, 1988), and HIV antibody testing is also offered in conjunction with many programs (e.g., Chitwood et al., 1990; Neaigus et al., 1990).

Although the majority of intervention programs have followed the pattern described above, some interventions have focused on encouraging peer support and mutual reinforcement among drug users for behaviors that reduce HIV/Acquired Human Immunodeficiency Syndrome (AIDS) risk (e.g., Carlson & Needle, 1989; Friedman, DeJong, & DesJarlais, 1988). In this approach, major emphasis is placed on recruiting members of the target population to serve as change agents and opinion leaders for the drug-using community at large. These programs aim at impacting drug users' social networks and eventually redefining social norms relating to practices that reduce HIV transmission risk. In a sense, the education and empowerment of individual drug users represents a means to the larger end of community social change.

Whether the focus of HIV/AIDS risk reduction efforts for drug users should be on the level of the individual or the social group cannot be answered simply. There are advantages and disadvantages to either approach, especially over the short term. Interventions oriented toward modifying the risk behaviors of a cohort of individuals from a drug-using population should be able to demonstrate larger changes in a shorter period of time compared with group-oriented interventions aimed primarily at influencing the broader social environment. Risk-behavior changes as a result of individual-oriented interventions, however, are likely to be restricted to those persons directly participating in the intervention, while the impact of group-oriented interventions should be more pervasive and may be more enduring and self-sustaining if the intervention is maintained initially over a sufficient period of time.

In practice, the effectiveness and efficiency of each strategy depends upon a variety of contextual and resource-related factors, only some of which can be determined with reasonable accuracy in a given situation. These factors include: (a) the number and diversity of individuals in the population of drug users targeted for intervention, (b) the variety and cohesiveness of their social networks, (c) the current level of awareness among individuals regarding HIV/AIDS and their experience with risk reduction methods, (d) the relative ease or difficulty of locating individuals and motivating them to participate in intervention sessions, (e) the relative ease or difficulty of motivating individuals to return for and/or participate in multiple intervention sessions, (f) the feasibility of engaging key members of social networks in the intervention process and maintaining ongoing contact with these individuals over a period of time, (g) the number and types of individuals comprising the intervention staff, and, finally, (h) the period of time over which it can be expected that the initial level of staffing for the intervention will be maintained and the estimated level and duration of subsequent staffing.

Owing to the indeterminate nature of many if not all of these factors in most settings, it would seem desirable that risk reduction interventions for drug users address both individual behavior change and social environment change simultaneously if at all possible. While a given intervention cannot in all likelihood be optimized for achievement of both of these goals, it may be feasible to optimize with respect to one goal while addressing the other goal to a lesser but meaningful degree.

A community-based HIV/AIDS risk reduction program for drug users characterized by this type of dual focus is currently being implemented in Long Beach, California, under a grant from the National Institute on Drug Abuse. The primary goal of this intervention is the facilitation of behavior change on the part of individual drug users who participate in the program. At the same time, there is a secondary goal and mechanism for influencing the broader social environment in which drug users function in terms of social norms and expectations regarding HIV/AIDS risk reduction. This paper describes the rationale and structure of the intervention program that has been developed and suggests possible pitfalls and implications.

BACKGROUND AND RATIONALE

The present intervention represents an outgrowth of an earlier individual counseling intervention conducted for injection drug users not in treatment in which behavioral contracting was utilized to facilitate definition and achievement of personal risk reduction goals (Corby, Rhodes, & Horn, 1991; Rhodes, Humfleet, & Corby, in press [a]). HIV testing was also provided, together with basic HIV/AIDS education and referrals. The core of the intervention consisted of a guided assessment of personal HIV risk, identification of achievable risk reduction goals for each client, personal contracting for goal attainment, and appraisal of goal progress and goal renegotiation. A special videotape entitled "Shooting Smart" was employed to increase participants' sense of personal vulnerability to HIV and their perception of the severity of HIV disease. This videotape featured HIV-positive Intravenous Drug Users (IDUs) from the local community in various stages of HIV infection who described how they became infected through sharing needles and the impact that HIV/AIDS had on their lives. Scenes of persons in the advanced stages of AIDS with highly visible symptoms were also included. The intervention was comprised of four individual counseling sessions, the first two of which were devoted to HIV testing, basic HIV/AIDS education, and bleach and condom skills training. The final two sessions were focused on personal goal setting and behavioral contracting as described above. The intervention was found to be effective in significantly reducing needle and, to a lesser extent, sexual risk of HIV infection in a sample of approximately 750 injection drug users (Rhodes, Humfleet, & Corby, in press [b]). In particular, the enhanced four-session intervention was superior to a two-session program consisting of basic HIV/AIDS education with HIV testing and counseling.

Drawing on this experience, a broader intervention was developed targeting crack cocaine as well as injection drug users. While this intervention retained structured behavioral counseling as a core, it increased the level of staff contact with participants and incorporated an explicit mechanism for providing ongoing social support for participants' behavior change activities. In addition, it was determined that counseling and skills training would be conducted in both group and individual formats instead of exclusively one-on-one.

The resulting Peer-supported AIDS Intervention for Risk Reduction (PAIRR) incorporates two individual sessions devoted to HIV-antibody testing and basic AIDS education, followed by two group workshop sessions plus an additional individual counseling session addressing salient behavior change issues. Content areas include (a) committing to change, (b) defining personal goals, (c) understanding stages of change, (d) implementing a plan of change, and (e) obtaining social support for personal change. Upon completion of these structured activities, participants are encouraged to attend informal monthly meetings for the next four to six months with a supportive peer they have previously identified. In addition, outreach workers maintain personal contacts with participants on a regular basis for the duration of the intervention.

A group of related behavioral models, constructs, and techniques formed the theoretical foundation for the PAIRR program. These included paradigms oriented specifically to the change of health-related behaviors as well as more general models of behavioral learning and motivation. Together, these provided a comprehensive framework for the development of specific intervention strategies likely to be successful in changing the HIV risk behaviors of drug users not in treatment. The health belief model and the related theory of protection motivation, together with Prochaska and Di-Clemente's (1983, 1986) stage model of behavior change, constituted the core framework for the intervention. The general behavioral/motivational models of social learning theory, social support, the theory of reasoned action, personal empowerment and self-efficacy, and behavioral contracting were influential in defining specific intervention strategies and program activities. The basic elements of these models and how each was utilized in the design of the present intervention are described below.

Health Belief Model and Protection-Motivation Theory

In the health belief model (Becker, 1974), an individual's beliefs regarding his/her own susceptibility to a specific disease and the perceived severity of that disease combine with risk-reduction benefits and barriers in determining whether protective health measures will be adopted by the individual. Protection motivation theory (Maddux & Rogers, 1983) likewise recognizes the importance of personal vulnerability and disease severity, and considers these together as defining the perceived magnitude of a particular health threat. Protection-motivation theory also stresses the importance of the individual's perception of the effectiveness of available risk-reduction options (similar to perceived benefits in the health belief model) as well as his or her sense of personal power to initiate and implement risk reduction activities (related to perceived barriers in the health belief model).

These core elements common to both theories constitute the foundation of the present intervention for injection drug and crack users. In the PAIRR program, specific activities focus on personalization of HIV/AIDS threat, evaluation of costs and benefits of HIV/AIDS risk reduction, and strategies for enhancing self-efficacy and overcoming barriers to change.

Stages of Behavioral Change

Prochaska and DiClemente (1983, 1986) have proposed a five-stage model of behavior change to describe the steps and processes associated with modification of problematic health behaviors. The model postulates distinct stages through which individuals pass in the course of changing their behavior: (a) precontemplation, (b) contemplation, (c) decision, (d) action, and (e) maintenance. Research in the areas of smoking cessation, weight control, dietary fat restriction, and alcohol and drug abuse support the model's utility in describing and understanding the process of health behavior change (Curry, Kristal, & Bowen, 1992; DiClemente & Hughes, 1990; Prochaska & DiClemente, 1986).

Movement through the five stages specified in the model is not necessarily monotonic, since many people fail in their initial attempts at change and revert temporarily to an earlier stage before moving forward again. Transition from stage to stage is mediated by stage-specific processes of change, which represent the strategies and techniques that individuals utilize in their attempts to deal with problem behaviors. Thus, the exercise of particular coping skills may be highly relevant for persons in the action and maintenance stages but not for individuals in earlier stages. The model also recognizes other influences affecting personal change that vary in importance at different places on the stage continuum. These are: (a) perceived pros versus cons for initiating change, (b) self-efficacy to implement change, and (c) temptation for relapse.

In the present intervention for drug users, the Prochaska model is employed as vehicle for increasing participants' understanding and clarifying their expectations regarding the process of personal behavior change. It is emphasized that individuals need a definite plan for implementing change, that change occurs in incremental steps rather than all at once, and that it is natural for people to experience problems and to relapse from time to time. In addition, when they first enter the program, participants are assisted in identifying their current stage of change in adopting behaviors that will protect them from HIV/AIDS. Throughout their involvement in the PAIRR program, the five-stage model serves as a metaphor for describing and interpreting participants' progress toward achievement of the personal risk-reduction goals they have defined.

Social Learning Theory

Social learning theory (Bandura, 1986, 1977a) emphasizes observational learning as the primary mechanism for acquisition of skills and behaviors in humans. Observational learning occurs through observing and copying the behavior of others, who are said to be modeling the behavior being learned. The role of reinforcement in social learning is also paramount–behaviors must be reinforced to be acquired and maintained. According to social learning theory, the learner can be reinforced vicariously through observing a model being rewarded for appropriate behavior. The learner may also be reinforced by direct praise or approval from the model or other source. Self-reinforcement, representing the learner's satisfaction in correctly performing a behavior being learned, is another reward mechanism considered by social learning theory.

Modeling in the context of AIDS risk reduction means that protective behaviors should be demonstrated or explained by persons who have themselves successfully adopted these behaviors. This is accomplished in the PAIRR program through role model stories describing drug users in the local community who have successfully changed their behavior to reduce HIV/AIDS risk. A different individual will model each type of risk reduction behavior, e.g, cleaning needles, using condoms, etc. Some individuals will tell their story in person; in other instances these will be videotaped.

Social Support

Social support from significant others, including one's spouse or peers, is also an important mechanism for reinforcing new behaviors. Personal change occurs in a context of social relationships, which, depending on their nature, can facilitate or undermine individual efforts at change (Bandura, 1990). The positive effects of social support have been widely researched. Wortman and Dunkel-Schetter (1987) point out that research on social support indicates positive effects for a variety of outcomes, including physical health, social functioning, and mental health. Social support is a critical component of many health-related behavior-change efforts. Ritter (1988) reports that social networks have been found to influence a variety of health-related behaviors and suggests that interventions should provide key network members with health-related information in order to increase the probability of preventive health behaviors. Research specifically examining HIV-related behaviors has found that peer support is strongly associated with risk reduction for injection drug users (Friedman, DesJarlais et al., 1987).

The present project assists the participants in the identification and development of support resources and encourages the involvement of support network members in the informal intervention activities. During the formal intervention sessions, participants identify potential sources of support for behavior change and discuss methods of obtaining support from others. Participants also are encouraged to bring a family member, significant other, or friend to informal support socials in order to link changes made in the intervention setting to the drug users' personal support networks.

Theory of Reasoned Action

Fishbein and Ajzen's (1975) theory of reasoned action views persuasive health communications as attempts to alter primary beliefs about the relationship between specific behaviors (e.g., condom use) and their consequences (e.g., reduced risk of HIV infection). According to this model, intentions to perform a recommended behavior depend on three factors: (a) beliefs as to the likelihood of particular consequences as a result of performing the behavior, (b) beliefs regarding the positive or negative nature of these consequences, and (c) beliefs about what others think one should do concerning performance of the behavior.

The theory of reasoned action is concerned with outcome value and probability of outcome occurrence as a function of presently held beliefs, attitudes, and values of individuals. An important element of the theory lies in the approach taken in specifying attitudes, beliefs, and target behaviors. The theory states that, in order for a measured attitude to predict behavior, the attitude must be narrowly and explicitly defined so that it closely relates and corresponds to the behavior in question, both in terms of context and specificity. This implies that, if one seeks to modify attitudes or beliefs so as to influence the likelihood of a behavior, the manipulation should directly address the specific cognitions that relate to the specific target behaviors. Attempts to modify global attitudes or beliefs apart from the behavioral context in which they are manifested will fail, it is stated, in terms of causing significant changes in specific target behaviors.

These principles are utilized in the present intervention in three ways. First, both the formal and informal activities of the program are oriented to enhance participants' perception that HIV/AIDS risk reduction is supported by other drug users like themselves. Second, the general structure of the intervention serves to increase the positive affect of participants toward performing risk reduction behaviors. Finally, participants are encouraged to consider the personal costs and benefits of specific HIV risk-reduction behaviors in the context of goal-related exercises.

Self-Efficacy and Personal Empowerment

Bandura's (1977b) self-efficacy and the concept of personal empowerment (Rappaport, 1987) are closely related constructs that emphasize the importance of perceived personal control as a determiner of coping style and outcomes. The comprehensive framework of self-efficacy asserts that the perception of personal power or efficacy in a problem situation determines whether an individual will try to cope with the problem, as well as how hard and for how long the individual will persevere in the face of setbacks and obstacles. In the model, a person's expectation of self-efficacy with respect to a given activity derives from four principal sources: (a) actual past performance, (b) vicarious experience with the activity, (c) verbal persuasion as to efficacy, (d) and experience of physiological arousal, e.g., anxiety. Perceived self-efficacy is seen as crucial to the adoption and satisfactory performance of protective health behaviors.

Personal empowerment may be defined as a global process in the course of which individuals develop a high degree of perceived autonomy and control in their social relationships and their relationships with institutions. The empowered individual is one who has high self-esteem, possesses a strong internal locus of control (Rotter, 1966), does not demonstrate learned helplessness (Abramson, Seligman, & Teasdale, 1984), and possesses an optimistic explanatory style for attribution of negative events (Alloy, Peterson, Abramson, & Seligman, 1984). Empowerment can also refer to enablement of individuals with respect to specific activities or behaviors such as those associated with HIV risk reduction.

In the present intervention, self-efficacy and personal empowerment issues are addressed within the context of activities related to goal-definition and refinement, identification and removal of barriers, development of risk-reduction skills and knowledge.

Behavioral Contracting

Behavioral or personal contracting is rooted in clinical practice, specifically behavior therapy and behavior modification (O'Banion & Whaley, 1981; Tharp & Wetzel, 1969). The technique has been employed extensively in the context of individual as well as group therapy, and it has been used with a variety of addictive behaviors, including overeating, smoking, and alcohol and drug use (Krasnegor, 1979; Stitzer, Bigelow, & McCaul, 1983). In recent years, personal contracting has been employed with patients in methadone maintenance programs as a means of reducing illicit drug use and facilitating other desirable behaviors (Dolan, Black, Penk, Robinowitz, & Deford, 1985, 1986; Magura, Casriel, Goldsmith, & Lipton, 1987). In personal contracting, an informal agreement is established with an individual defining a particular behavioral goal that is to be achieved within a specified period of time. It has been suggested by O'Banion and Whaley (1981) that three factors have an important bearing on the extent to which behavioral agreements will be upheld: (a) the exactness with which the desired behavior has been specified, (b) how frequently and accurately the target behavior can be observed, and (c) how effectively and consistently reinforcement is applied.

Elements of behavioral contracting are employed in the PAIRR program to increase the likelihood that participants will achieve their personal risk-reduction goals. The intervention emphasizes exact specification of behavioral goals, time frames for accomplishing specific steps, and meaningful reinforcement for behavior-change efforts.

INTERVENTION STRUCTURE

A general description of the intervention is described in the previous section. This section provides a brief description of Sessions One and Two, which are described in greater detail in the National Institute on Drug Abuse (1992) intervention manual. A detailed outline, description, and goals for Sessions Three through Five are provided, as well as a description of the informal supportive activities.

Session One (Individual)

The goals of Session One are to provide basic HIV transmission and prevention information, modeling of risk reduction methods, and counseling about HIV-antibody testing. During this session, counselors provide information on the HIV disease spectrum, modes of transmission, and methods of reducing HIV risks. Demonstrations are conducted on the correct methods of needle cleaning and condom use. Counselors also describe the HIV-antibody testing process, potential test results, and implications of those results. Participants are then offered testing.

Session Two (Individual)

The goals of Session Two are to provide HIV-antibody testing results, reinforcement of HIV-related knowledge, and augmentation of HIV prevention skills. Testing results are provided at the beginning of the session. Participants are allowed time to react and are encouraged to verbalize their feelings. Exact meanings of the test results are reviewed. In order to reinforce knowledge, HIV transmission and prevention methods are reviewed. During this review, the participant is asked to demonstrate the correct procedures for needle cleaning and condom use. This demonstration by the participant along with corrective feedback from the counselor serves to augment the skills of the participant.

Session Three (Group)

The goals of Session Three are to: (a) introduce participants and facilitator(s), (b) provide a brief overview of the intervention goals, activities, and ground rules, (c) reinforce the personal relevance of HIV/AIDS risk and personal vulnerability, (d) review specific risk behaviors and risk reduction methods, (e) provide practical information on the sequence of steps in changing personal behavior, and (f) underline the influence of social support on behavior change.

The discussion of personal vulnerability and the relevance of risk reduction is facilitated through a group exercise in which group members are asked whether they know or have heard of anyone with HIV/AIDS in the local community. No identifying information can be shared during this exercise. The facilitator utilizes the information provided by participants to highlight that HIV infection is occurring in the participants' community. In addition, the facilitator shares local HIV statistics with the group members, emphasizing the impact of HIV in the injection drug using community.

Following this, the facilitator leads an exercise which requires group members to identify HIV transmission routes and risk reduction methods. Sex, drug, and needle risk behaviors as well as preventive measures are always included in this review. At the end of this group exercise, a form is distributed to group members which lists a series of risk behaviors. Participants are asked to rate themselves on each particular risk behavior in order to re-examine their personal risk(s).

The remainder of this session focuses on two theoretical concepts important to behavior change. Through a didactic presentation, the facilitator provides information on the sequence of steps typically experienced in changing personal behavior (stages of behavioral change). This information is conveyed by sharing the story of a drug user who attempts to quit using drugs. The story encompasses each step of the behavioral change process. Following this story, participants are asked to identify which step best describes their current personal status in regard to various risk reduction methods, e.g., cleaning needles, reducing number of sex partners, etc.

At this point, the importance and influence of social support in behavior change is introduced. This discussion is facilitated by describing a scenario in which an injector wants to change his/her behavior but no one in his/her peer group is supportive of that change. Participants respond to this scenario and identify how the change process might be facilitated. Group members are then asked to identify someone within their personal network of friends/family who has previously provided support and to describe how that support helped or hindered their attempts at change. At the end of this session, participants are prompted to consider individuals in their support network who would encourage and be supportive of their efforts to reduce personal HIV risks.

Session Four (Group)

The goals of Session Four are: (a) overview of the goal development process, (b) definition of a personal goal by each participant, (c) discussion of barriers to personal goals, (d) discussion of methods for overcoming barriers, and (e) exposure to role models who have been successful at risk reduction.

The overview of the goal development process is provided through the review of two "model" goals. Initially the facilitator discusses the general guidelines for setting a goal, i.e., it should be specific, it should be realistic, it should be short-term, etc. Then the facilitator reviews, with active group evaluation, examples of well-developed and poorly developed goals. Group members are then asked to define an area of behavior change, e.g., needle sharing, bleaching, or condom use, as well as a short-term goal. These goals are shared with the group and discussed. Utilizing the personal goals defined by the group members, potential barriers to goal achievement and means of overcoming barriers are discussed. Participants are prompted to provide feedback/suggestions to other group members and these suggestions are utilized by participants to refine their goal(s).

After goals have been defined, peer support for behavior change is discussed. Participants are asked whether they were able to identify a supportive individual(s) since the initial discussion in Session Three and, if so, to share this information with the group. Participants are then asked if this is a person who could be supportive of the goal behavior they have just identified for themselves. If not, alternatives are discussed.

As a means of enhancing the commitment and self-efficacy of group members, role models participate in the final segment of Session Four. These models share information about their personal risk reduction experience, describing their attempts at change, problems encountered, and success experiences. The presentations are conducted by participants of the previous Long Beach educational intervention who have been successful in reducing their HIV/AIDS risk in a variety of ways. Role model success stories encompass five risk reduction behaviors including: (a) stopping drug use, (b) not sharing needles or works, (c) always bleaching needles or works, (d) using condoms consistently, and (e) decreasing number of sex partners. These success stories can be presented by either the live model or through a video format.

Session Five (Individual)

The goals of Session Five are: (a) review of the participant's personal goal, (b) discussion of potential support resources and methods for eliciting that support, (c) identification of at least one supportive peer, and (d) discussion of support socials and future contacts. All activities in this session are conducted in an individual format.

At the beginning of the session, the counselor and participant review the goal(s) established during Session Four. This provides an opportunity for the additional refinement of goal(s), if necessary. After reviewing the goal(s) of the participant, the individual is asked to identify potential sources of support for HIV/AIDS risk reduction efforts. Once potential resources are identified, methods of obtaining support from others are discussed. Role plays focusing on how to engage support for behavior change may be utilized to increase the individual's sense of personal efficacy.

After identification of potential support resources and discussion of methods for eliciting support, individuals are asked to identify at least one person in their support network who they will enlist to help them change their behavior over the next several months. Participants are encouraged to invite this individual(s) to the support socials following completion of the intervention. Prior to concluding the session, there is a discussion of follow-up activities and an overview of future contacts/activities. These activities include: (a) attending monthly support socials, (b) contact in two weeks with outreach worker to determine success in soliciting support, and (c) other ongoing contacts with the project, e.g., food bank, drug treatment referral, etc.

Monthly Support Groups

Monthly support groups are offered for participants following completion of workshop sessions. These groups, envisioned as support socials, are held at various locations in the community that have been identified as providing easy access for participants. Each event lasts approximately two hours and includes a meal. Participants are encouraged to bring the supportive peer(s) they have identified during the previous contacts to every support group. In addition, participants are invited to bring other individuals from their support network as well. If individuals are unable to identify a supportive peer during the intervention, an effort is made to link them to other participants from their community during the monthly support group meetings.

Although informal, each support social includes a brief structured segment dealing with HIV/AIDS risk reduction. During this time, behavior change activities are reinforced and validated, and the important role played by support buddies is recognized. In addition, project staff encourage participants and their companion(s) on an individual level as they mingle during the event. Each participant attends a minimum of two support events during the five-month period following completion of the intervention. Telephone contacts and personal visits by outreach workers are utilized to encourage participation in support groups.

Outreach Worker Supportive Interactions

Each participant in the enhanced intervention is assigned to a specific outreach worker, who has responsibility for maintaining contact with the participant to ensure insofar as possible that all intervention sessions are completed and that at least two support socials are attended. Outreach workers are required to document a minimum of two face-to-face contacts with each participant, in addition to contacts occurring at scheduled activities, during the period of the intervention. There is a goal of having five total support-group and outreach-worker contacts combined for each participant, in addition to workshop attendance.

DISCUSSION

The Personal AIDS Intervention Risk-Reduction program has been structured to address the issues of both injection drug and crack cocaine users who are not currently in drug treatment. Injection users have a primary needle-use risk for HIV and also, potentially, a secondary risk arising from sexual behavior. Crack users, on the other hand, have sexual behavior as their primary, and only direct, HIV risk factor. In terms of HIV risk-reduction behaviors, this implies condom use and reduction of the number of sex partners as the only common denominator for both groups. It is also possible to promote drug abstinence as a risk-reduction for both types of drug users, but it is recognized that this is directly related to HIV risk only for injection users. As indicated earlier, the changes that have been observed in sexual practices among injection drug users following participation in HIV interventions have been considerably smaller than the changes related to needle risk. Whether this is because sex risk is relatively less salient among individuals who have a primary HIV risk associated with their drug use or because changes in sexual behavior are problematic in general is not known. In either case, this phenomenon has significant implications for the success of HIV risk-reduction efforts among crack cocaine users.

The PAIRR intervention will be provided to HIV-seropositive as well as to seronegative individuals. HIV transmission issues and personal behaviors are the same for both groups, and risk-reduction messages can be made applicable to either situation with little difficulty. Some adjustment of intervention content will be necessary, however, primarily in the workshop sessions to recognize seropositive individuals' special perspective and to protect their confidentiality. It is important to include seropositive individuals in the efficacy study in order to be able to demonstrate explicitly that the intervention is appropriate and effective for persons who are already infected with HIV.

An intervention of the type described requires an indigenous outreach staff capable of recruiting and maintaining contact with program participants over a period of time. The success of all programs targeting drug users who are not enrolled in drug treatment rests in large measure with the effectiveness of the outreach effort and the expertise of outreach staff. It is important always to bear this fact in mind in developing HIV/AIDS intervention programs for this population.

REFERENCES

Abramson, L. Y., Seligman, M. E. P., & Teasdale, J. D. (1978). Learned helplessness in humans: Critique and reformulation. *Journal of Abnormal Psychology*, *87*, 49-74.

Alloy, L. B., Peterson, C., Abramson, L. Y., & Seligman, M. E. (1984). Attributional and the generality of learned helplessness. *Journal of Personality and Social Psychology*, *46*, 681-687.

Bandura, A. (1990). Perceived self-efficacy in the exercise of control over AIDS infection. *Evaluation and Program Planning*, *13*, 9-17.

Bandura, A. (1986). *Social foundations of thought and action: A social cognitive theory.* Englewood Cliffs, NJ: Prentice Hall.

Bandura, A. (1977a). *Social learning theory.* Englewood Cliffs, NJ: Prentice-Hall.

Bandura, A. (1977b). Self-efficacy: Toward a unifying theory of behavioral change. *Psychological Review*, *84*, 191-215.

Becker, M. H. (1974). The health belief model and personal health behavior. *Health Education Monographs*, *2*, 324-508.

Bruneau, J., Brabant, M., Lamothe, F., Soto, J., Vincelette, J., & Fauvel, M. (1991, June). *Reported behavior changes in a cohort of injection drug users (IDUs) in Montreal.* Paper presented at the Seventh International Conference on AIDS, Florence, Italy.

Carlson, G., & Needle, R. (1989). *Sponsoring addict self-organization (addicts against AIDS): A case study.* Paper presented at the First Annual National AIDS Demonstration Research Conference, Rockville, MD.

Chitwood, D. D., McCoy, C. B., McCoy, H. V., McKay, C., McBride, D. C., & Comerford, M. (1990, June). *Evaluation of a risk reduction program for intravenous drug users.* Paper presented at Sixth International Conference on AIDS, San Francisco.

Corby, N. H., Rhodes, F., & Horn, J. (1991). Enhanced AIDS prevention counseling for injection drug users incorporating high-threat appeals and personal contracting In *Proceedings of the First Annual NADR Meeting.* Rockville, MD: National Institute on Drug Abuse.

Curry, S. J., Kristal, A. R., & Bowen, D. J. (1992). An application of the stage model of behavior change to dietary fat reduction. *Health Education Research*, *7*, 97-105.

DiClemente, C. C., & Hughes, S. O. (1990). Stages and profiles in outpatient alcoholism treatment. *Journal of Substance Abuse*, *2*, 217-235.

Dolan, M. P., Black, J. L., Penk, W. E., Robiniwitz, R., & Deford, H. A. (1985). Contracting for treatment termination to reduce illicit drug use among methadone maintenance treatment failures. *Journal of Consulting and Clinical Psychology, 53*, 549-551.

Dolan, M. P., Black, J. L., Penk, W. E., Robiniwitz, R., & Deford, H. A. (1986). Predicting the outcome of contingency contracting for drug abuse. *Behavior Therapy, 68*, 485-493.

Fishbein, M., & Ajzen, I. (1975). *Belief, attitude, and behavior: An introduction to theory and research.* Reading, MA: Addison-Wesley.

Friedman, S. R., DesJarlais, D. C., Sotheran, J. L., Garber, J., Cohen, H., & Smith, D. (1987). AIDS and self-organization among intravenous drug users. *International Journal of the Addictions, 22*, 201-220.

Friedman, S. R., DeJong, W. M., & DesJarlais, D. C. (1988). Problems and dynamics of organizing intravenous drug users for AIDS prevention. *Health Education Research, 3*(1), 49-57.

Iguchi, M. Y., Watters, J., & Biernacki, P. (1990). Update: Reducing HIV transmission in intravenous drug users not in drug treatment–United States. *Morbidity & Mortality Weekly Report, 39*, 529, 535-538.

Krasnegor, N. A. (Ed.). (1979). *Behavioral analysis and treatment of substance abuse.* Rockville, MD: National Institute on Drug Abuse.

Liebman, J., Bowden, J., Meredith, L., & Mulia, N. (1990, October). Individual and group counseling and education to promote HIV risk reduction among intravenous drug users and their sex partners. Paper presented at annual meeting of the American Public Health Association, New York.

Liebman, J., McIlvaine, D. S., Kotranski, L., & Lewis, R. (1990). AIDS prevention for IV drug users and their sexual partners in Philadelphia. *American Journal of Public Health, 80*, 615-616.

Maddux, J. E., & Rogers, R. W. (1983). Protection motivation theory and self-efficacy: A revised theory of fear appeals and attitude change. *Journal of Experimental Social Psychology, 19*, 469-479.

Magura, S., Casriel, C., Goldsmith, D. S., & Lipton, D. S. (1987). Contracting with clients in methadone treatment. *Journal of Contemporary Social Work, 68*, 485-493.

Moss, A. R., & Chaisson, R. (1988). AIDS and intravenous drug use in San Francisco. *AIDS and Public Policy, 3*, 37-41.

National AIDS Research Consortium (1990). Risk behaviors for HIV transmission among intravenous drug users not in drug treatment–United States, 1987-1989. *Morbidity & Mortality Weekly Report, 39*, 273-276.

National Institute on Drug Abuse (1992). *The NIDA standard intervention model for injection drug users not in treatment: Intervention manual.* Rockville, MD: National Institute on Drug Abuse.

Neaigus, A., Sufian, M., Friedman, S. R., Goldsmith, D. S., Stepherson, B., Mota, P., Pascal, J., & Des Jarlais, D. C. (1990). Effects of outreach intervention on risk reduction among intravenous drug users. *AIDS Education and Prevention, 2*, 253-271.

O'Banion, D. R., & Whaley, D. L. (1981). *Behavior contracting: Arranging contingencies of reinforcement.* New York: Springer Publishing Co.

Prochaska, J. O., & DiClemente, C. C. (1983). Stages and processes of self-change in smoking: Towards an integrative model of change. *Journal of Consulting and Clinical Psychology, 51*, 390-395.

Prochaska, J. O., & DiClemente, C. C. (1986). Toward a comprehensive model of change. In W. Miller & N. Heather (Ed.), *Treating addictive behaviors* (pp. 3-27). New York: Plenum Press.

Rappaport, J. (1987). Terms of empowerment/exemplars of prevention: Toward a theory of community psychology. *American Journal of Community Psychology, 15*, 121-148.

Ritter, C. (1988). Social supports, social networks, and health behaviors. In D. Gochman (Ed.), *Health behavior: Emerging perspectives* (pp. 149-161). New York: Plenum Press.

Rhodes, F., Humfleet, G. L., & Corby, N. H. (in press [a]). Efficacy of alternative counseling strategies on AIDS risk reduction among IDUs: Preliminary findings. In *Proceedings of the Second Annual NADR Meeting.* Rockville, MD: National Institute on Drug Abuse.

Rhodes, F., Humfleet, G. L., & Corby, N. H. (in press [b]). Effects of individual counseling interventions on AIDS risk behaviors of injection drug users. In *Proceedings of the Third Annual NADR Meeting.* Rockville, MD: National Institute on Drug Abuse.

Rotter, J. B. (1966). Generalized expectancies for internal versus external control of reinforcement. *Psychological Monographs, 80*, (1, Whole No. 609).

Stitzer, M. L., Bigelow, G. E., & McCaul, M. E. (1983). Behavioral approaches to drug abuse. In M. Hersen (Ed.), *Progress in Behavior Modification* (Vol. 14, pp. 49-123). New York: Academic Press.

Tharp, R. G., & Wetzel, R. J. (1969). *Behavioral modification in the natural environment.* New York: Academic Press.

Tross, S., Abdul-Quadar, A. S., Silvert, H. M., Rapkin, B., Des Jarlais, D. C., & Friedman, S. (1991, June). Determinants of needle sharing change in street recruited New York City IV drug users. Paper presented at the Seventh International Conference on AIDS, Florence, Italy.

Wortman, C. B., & Dunkel-Schetter, C. (1987). Conceptual and methodological issues in the study of social support. In A. Baum & J.E. Singer (Eds.), *Handbook of psychology and health* (pp. 63-108). Hillsdale, NJ: Lawrence Erlbaum Associates.

An Office-Based AIDS Prevention Program for High Risk Drug Users

Jon Liebman, MS
Nina Mulia, MPH

SUMMARY. There is an urgent need to develop effective AIDS prevention programs to assist high-risk individuals to change their behavior. This article describes an office-based intervention program for out-of-treatment injection drug users (IDUs) and crack cocaine users recruited from street settings in a major urban area. The relationships of program elements to key aspects of the Health Belief Model and Social Learning Theory are discussed, as are operational considerations of working with this population in a non-treatment setting.

INTRODUCTION

As the Acquired Immune Deficiency Syndrome (AIDS) epidemic continues its worldwide spread without the prospect of either an

Jon Liebman and Nina Mulia are Senior Research Associates with Philadelphia Health Management Corporation, 260 South Broad Street, Philadelphia, PA 19102-5085.

The authors gratefully acknowledge the contributions of Joanne Bowden and other staff of PHMC's AIDS Prevention Project.

This project has been supported by the National Institute on Drug Abuse, grants DA06919 and DA04841.

[Haworth co-indexing entry note:] "An Office-Based AIDS Prevention Program for High Risk Drug Users." Liebman, Jon, and Nina Mulia. Co-published simultaneously in *Drugs & Society* (The Haworth Press, Inc.) Vol. 7, No. 3/4, 1993, pp. 205-223; and: *AIDS and Community-Based Drug Intervention Programs: Evaluation and Outreach* (ed: Dennis G. Fisher, and Richard Needle) The Haworth Press, Inc., 1993, pp. 205-223. Multiple copies of this article/chapter may be purchased from The Haworth Document Delivery Center [1-800-3-HAWORTH; 9:00 a.m. - 5:00 p.m. (EST)].

Copyright © 1993 by Taylor & Francis

effective vaccine or cure in the near future, there is a compelling need to develop effective prevention programs to assist individuals to reduce their risk of infection with Human Immunodeficiency Virus (HIV). This need is particularly acute for drug users, who are at extremely high risk of acquiring and transmitting HIV infection through unprotected sex and the sharing of contaminated injection equipment. As of April, 1992 injection drug users (IDUs) represented 29% of all adult and adolescent AIDS cases in the United States (CDC, 1992). The AIDS epidemic among IDUs is also tightly linked to the spread of the epidemic in the larger, non-IDU population, as many IDUs engage in sexual relations with non-IDUs (Brown & Primm, 1988; Chitwood, McCoy & Comerford, 1990; Liebman, Mulia & McIlvaine, 1992; Murphy, 1988; Rhodes et al., 1990). Fifty-three percent of all adult and adolescent AIDS cases acquired through heterosexual contact involved sex with an IDU, and 58% of all pediatric cases were associated with a mother who was an IDU or the sex partner of an IDU (CDC, 1992). Moreover, there is growing evidence that the national epidemic of crack cocaine use may be associated with the rapid spread of HIV and other sexually transmitted diseases (STDs), due to the high frequency of unprotected sex among crack users (Rolfs, Goldberg & Sharrar, 1990; Minkoff et al., 1990; Mellinger et al., 1991).

AIDS prevention efforts directed at drug users outside of treatment settings have generally fallen into three categories: mass media campaigns, targeted outreach efforts and office-based interventions. Mass media programs directed at drug users have attempted to reach them as part of a broader audience to provide basic information about AIDS and its prevention, including exhortations to abstain from sharing needles, and more generally, from drug use. Targeted outreach programs have attempted to selectively reach high risk drug users in community settings, delivering prevention messages through face-to-face interactions, distributing condoms and bleach kits, and, in some locations, distributing sterile needles; some have also actively encouraged participation in drug treatment (Jackson, Rotkiewicz & Baxter, 1990; Mason, 1990). Office-based interventions have been developed in numerous cities as part of the National AIDS Demonstration Research (NADR) program sponsored by the National Institute on Drug Abuse (NIDA) and other initiatives. These typically include one or more sessions of individual and/or group counseling and education, HIV antibody testing and referrals for other services.

These efforts have succeeded in raising the level of AIDS awareness among drug users and encouraging a significant portion of them to reduce their risk behavior to some degree (Chaisson, Osmond, Moss, Feldman & Biernacki, 1987; Iguchi et al., 1990; McAuliffe et al., 1987). More effective efforts are needed, however, as needle sharing and unprotected sex remain common practices and the incidence of HIV infection remains high. Unfortunately, although the field of health education is well established, there is little literature of a practical nature to guide service providers in the development of AIDS prevention programs for drug users who are not willing to enter treatment. This paper attempts to fill that gap by describing an office-based model for conducting AIDS prevention with out-of-treatment IDUs and crack cocaine users in one community of Philadelphia. Specifically, we address the project's background; the relevant health education theory used in developing this intervention program; and how this theory is operationalized, including practical considerations of conducting such work with a difficult, non-compliant and occasionally dangerous population.

BACKGROUND

In the spring of 1988 Philadelphia Health Management Corporation (PHMC) initiated a street outreach project targeting IDUs in North Philadelphia, the city's most active area for drug selling and use. Soon after, office-based individual and group education and counseling activities were added, as was HIV antibody testing. As is described elsewhere (Liebman, McIlvaine, Kotranski, & Lewis, 1990; Liebman, Mulia & Bowden, 1992), this effort demonstrated the ability to recruit IDUs from street settings and engage them repeatedly in individual and group sessions.

PHMC's AIDS prevention program was substantially revised in 1991. Crack users were targeted for intervention, as well as IDUs; outreach workers were redeployed to recruit a more demographically diverse population of drug users; the content and format of the office-based intervention was redesigned; and a more rigorous evaluation design was implemented. With these changes, the project became more grounded in health education theory, more accessible to out-of-treatment drug users, and placed greater emphasis on reducing sexual risk behavior.

THEORETICAL BASE FOR INTERVENTION ACTIVITIES

This revised office-based intervention has been based on two widely used theoretical models of health behavior change, the Health Belief Model (HBM) and Social Learning Theory (SLT). The office-based intervention has also been designed to complement the project's street outreach component, so that each reinforces the other.

The Health Belief Model (HBM) was originally developed by researchers at the Public Health Service to address problems of non-participation in health screenings, vaccination, and other short-term activities. The HBM has served as a theoretical basis for the design of numerous health promotion efforts, and its applicability to many different areas of health promotion has been demonstrated (Becker, 1974; Janz & Becker, 1984). As articulated by Rosenstock (1990), the original HBM attempts to explain health behavior as a function of an individual's perceptions of: (a) personal susceptibility to the illness or condition in question, (b) the severity of the illness or condition, (c) benefits of taking a particular action or modifying behavior, and (d) barriers to taking action. It was later recognized that the HBM did not adequately address the difficulties involved in making permanent changes in long established habits (Rosenstock, Strecher & Becker, 1988), and the model was expanded to include Bandura's concept of self-efficacy (1977), or "the conviction that one can successfully execute the behavior required to produce the outcomes." Together, the components of the model suggest that in order for individuals to alter their HIV-related risk behavior, they must believe in their own personal susceptibility to HIV infection and AIDS; believe that HIV infection will seriously and negatively affect their lives; believe that changing their behavior (e.g., using condoms and cleaning needles) will be effective in preventing HIV infection; believe that the benefits of these actions outweigh the expected costs or barriers (material, interpersonal, etc.); and believe in their own ability to initiate and sustain changes in their behavior.

The HBM suggests that interventions should be designed to affect the beliefs of individuals. Although this is a potentially effective approach, this focus on individual expectancies may be less applicable to AIDS prevention work with drug users. Janz and Becker caution, "... the HBM is a *psychosocial* model; as such it is limited to accounting for as much of the variance in individuals' health-related behaviors as can be explained by their attitudes and beliefs. It is clear that other forces influence health actions as well," including behaviors with "a substantial habitual component obviating any ongoing psychosocial decision-making process" (1984, p. 44). This is certainly the case for addicted individuals, whose behaviors are driven by physical as well as psychological habituation.

Social Learning Theory (SLT), a broad set of social-psychological constructs developed since the 1940's, addresses the processes by which individuals learn and alter their behavior. Central to SLT is the notion of a triadic relationship between individual behavior, the environment and a range of personal factors, particular cognitive abilities related to learning. Change in any one of these domains is assumed to affect the others in a reciprocal relationship. Rather than the HBM's focus on individual beliefs as predictors of an action or health behavior, SLT is concerned with a process by which individual factors affect and are in turn affected by both behaviors and the larger environment. As articulated by Perry, Baranowski and Parcel (1990), SLT encompasses several key concepts relevant to the design of health promotion programs. PHMC's intervention program draws principally on four of these: (a) "behavioral capacity," or the mastery of skills necessary to perform actions such as condom use and proper needle hygiene; (b) "observational learning," which refers to the capacity of an individual to learn by watching the actions of others and the consequences of those actions; (c) "self-efficacy," previously discussed in relation to the HBM; and (d) "emotional coping responses," referring to the development of strategies and skills for coping with stresses, such as pressures to engage in risk behavior.

The applicability of aspects of the HBM and SLT to AIDS prevention programs involving behavioral change is supported by several authors (DesJarlais & Friedman, 1988; Kelly, St. Lawrence, Hood & Brasfield, 1989; Sorenson, 1991). We have been particularly influenced by two specific approaches to behavioral change consistent with these theories: the use of credible models to deliver intervention messages, and the creation of peer support for risk reduction. The use of credible models, or individuals with whom project participants can identify in terms of life experiences, has been recognized as an important aspect of AIDS prevention work (Kelly et al., 1989; Magura, Shapiro, Grossman & Lipton, 1989; Fisher, 1988; Mays & Cochran, 1988) and is consistent with both the concepts of self-efficacy and observational learning. Bandura (1977) argues that through social comparison, successful risk reduction by individuals perceived to be similar to oneself can engender an enhanced sense of one's own ability to initiate behavioral change. Similarly, the creation of peer support through group intervention activities allows fellow participants to serve as credible models for each other, and to create an environment in which group pressure is a catalyst for behavioral change (Fisher, 1988).

Using this theoretical base, we have developed an intervention program which has four basic objectives. First, high risk individuals must acquire knowledge about HIV/AIDS and the desire to reduce their risk of infection. Working with marginalized individuals who are often poorly educated and lack access to reliable sources of information, we have implemented intensive outreach and other educational efforts to meet this need. Second, individuals must learn the manual skills needed to properly use condoms and bleach. In a society which has only recently permitted open discussion of condom use, but still does not support explicit public education about how to use one or how to clean injection equipment, AIDS prevention programs must provide high risk individuals the opportunity to develop proficient skills in condom use and needle sterilization so that they can comfortably practice these methods on their own. Third, the material means to protect oneself must be made available to high risk individuals. In our project this has meant the widespread distribution of condoms and bleach kits by outreach workers, while other programs have improved access to drug treatment services and distributed sterile needles. Lastly, individuals must be assisted in developing the inner and interpersonal resources to overcome barriers to adopting lower risk lifestyles. This includes raising beliefs of self-efficacy, improving the social skills needed to negotiate condom and bleach use and to avoid sharing injection equipment, and providing adequate support to initiate and maintain new behavioral patterns in the face of resistance from partners and peers.

PRACTICAL CONSIDERATIONS

Practical considerations are often of equal or greater importance than are theoretical ones in the design of community intervention programs, particularly when working with drug users who may be distrustful of the intentions of the project, non-compliant with program requirements, and potentially disruptive and physically threatening to project staff. Practical constraints on program design include both operational issues, affecting the ability of the project to reach and engage high risk individuals, and efficacy issues, concerning whether the intervention is designed to most effectively influence participants' risk behavior.

Five basic operational issues were considered in the design of the project. First, office-based activities are supported by the project's strong street outreach component. In working with this population in a non-institutional setting, street outreach has been essential not only to recruit individuals for participation in office-based counseling and education, but more fundamentally to build credibility and trust with the drug-using community. The on-going presence of project staff on the street, in shooting galleries and crack houses, and in other community settings has been essential to overcome fears that the project might be related to law enforcement agencies or other organizations hostile to drug users.

Second, the location of the field office was carefully considered. Because the project operates in a racially mixed (Black, White and Latino) but segregated area of the city, it has been critical to locate the field office on a major commercial street which is not perceived as belonging to any one racial/ethnic group. Were this not the case, it would be extremely difficult to recruit participants from different groups.

Third, incentives for participation were built into the project. In addition to the social and health benefits of participation, it has been important to the project's operational success to provide small financial and material incentives for participation. Participants receive personal care items, food, used clothing and small financial payments. Occasionally, special events are held for participants, such as an annual Thanksgiving dinner.

Fourth, the physical security of the office was addressed through careful consideration of the layout of the office, strict rules prohibiting staff from working alone in the office, and by hiring a security guard. The benefits of such actions extend to project participants, as well as staff. As one female participant explained, "I like coming here because it's the one place where I don't have to worry about nobody messing with me."

Lastly, the format of the program was designed so as to maximize its accessibility and acceptability to potential participants. Noncompliance in attending rigidly sequenced intervention activities must be expected, particularly when working with addicted individuals. To adapt the project to fit the lifestyle of participants, a modified drop-in format was adopted which allows participants to attend repeatedly without adhering to a strict sequencing of events.

Efficacy issues include those considerations which help present AIDS prevention messages in a context in which participants are most likely to respond to them. First, because the majority of participants in our project are struggling with multiple, immediate threats to their health and well-being, including homelessness, violence and extreme poverty, in addition to drug abuse, the intervention program includes discussion of these issues as they relate to AIDS risk behavior. Second, we have used a variety of techniques, including didactic methods, audiovisual programs, group discussions, role playing, and presentations by outside guests, including former drug users with AIDS, to enliven the presentation of material. Lastly, while trying to control the sequencing of events as little as possible (in the interests of accessibility) we have found it important to structure the intervention such that participants progress from individual to group interactions, from single-sex to mixed-gender groups, and from simple didactic teaching about HIV transmission and prevention to more complex interpersonal and experiential activities.

DESCRIPTION OF INTERVENTION ACTIVITIES

As shown in Figure 1, the intervention program consists of activities conducted in three distinct situations. Initial contact with potential program participants is made by the project's outreach staff, who approach individuals whom they suspect to be drug users on the streets and in other community settings. Outreach workers are selected to serve as credible models; almost all are from the communities in which they work and some are former drug users. They attempt to work with small social groups, as well as with isolated individuals, to encourage peer support for risk reduction. Outreach staff use didactic techniques to influence the beliefs of clients, conduct limited skills training in the use of condoms and bleach, and confront the environmental constraint of a lack of condoms and bleach by distributing these materials. Finally, outreach workers recruit IDUs and crack users for participation in the project's office-based activities, and maintain contact with them over the following months to encourage their retention in the project.

Approximately half of the IDUs and crack users referred by outreach workers actually present themselves at the field office. There, they meet individually with a health educator for a 30 to 60 minute counseling session, after first being interviewed to provide data for the project's research and evaluation components. At this individual counseling session, the health educator presents basic information about the biology and epidemiology of HIV, assists the participant to discuss his own risk behavior and to identify ways to reduce the risk of infection, and, using anatomical models and a syringe, demonstrates the use of condoms and bleach which the participant, in turn, is encouraged to rehearse. Referrals are made for participants in need of additional services, including AIDS-related case management, support groups, drug treatment, health care, and housing assistance. HIV antibody testing is discussed and pretest counseling provided to clarify what information may be learned

FIGURE 1.   PROGRAM COMPONENTS AND ACTIVITIES

STREET OUTREACH   Identification of high-risk drug users

                                AIDS prevention education

                                Brief counseling

                                Distribution of condoms and bleach kits

                                Recruitment for office-based activities

INDIVIDUAL COUNSELING   AIDS prevention education

(2 sessions)   Risk reduction counseling

                                HIV antibody counseling and testing

                                Referrals for services

GROUP SESSIONS

    Single-sex groups   4 Modules

    (up to 12 sessions)   Introduction to HIV/AIDS

                                Safer sex

                                Safer drug use

                                Barriers to risk reduction

    Mixed-gender sessions   Address individual and environmental/structural

    (up to 12 sessions)   issues related to HIV risk reduction

from testing, how the participant will use this information, and the potential risks involved. If desired, blood is drawn for HIV antibody testing at the end of the counseling session. All participants are encouraged to return within three weeks for a second individual counseling session. For those who have had blood drawn, this session is used to provide test results with appropriate counseling, and to develop a plan of action for HIV-infected individuals.

Project participants are strongly encouraged to attend group sessions in the weeks following their individual counseling sessions at the field office. Two kinds of group sessions are conducted: single-sex sessions addressing basic AIDS prevention issues, and mixed-gender sessions addressing more complex interpersonal and structural issues related to risk reduction. Single-sex sessions consist of a four-module series held on a rotating, four week schedule. Participants are encouraged to attend as many as 12 single-sex sessions over a six month period, and must attend at least 3 sessions before they can attend a mixed-gender group. Previous experience has shown that the single-sex groups are a better setting for introducing the sensitive topics involved in AIDS prevention and to allow participants to adjust to discussing sexual behavior with others before doing so with members of the opposite sex. In addition, the four modules provide a basic introduction to AIDS (even for those participants who do not attend all four modules) that serves as a foundation for the more in-depth discussion and experiential activities of the mixed-gender groups.

The first single-sex module presents introductory information on HIV and AIDS, including AIDS epidemiology and transmission, effects of HIV on the immune system, and symptoms of HIV-related illness. Didactic techniques are used to present information and to correct participants' misperceptions. Videotapes and other visual displays are used, as are participatory exercises. When available, recovering addicts with AIDS and other relevant guests talk about their experiences before and after infection with HIV.

The second single-sex module concentrates on safer sex issues, including infection and re-infection with HIV and STDs through specific sex acts, differences between the many STDs, risk reduction methods, and barriers and strategies to adopting safer sexual practices. Safer sex methods are demonstrated and participants practice using condoms, spermicide and dental dams on anatomical models. "Safer sex kits" which include these materials are distributed. Participants are asked to share their personal reasons for not using barrier protection and to identify problems in communication with partners around safer sex. Role plays are used to develop better communication skills, to give participants practice in dealing with stressful situations and to stimulate group discussion.

The third module focuses on addiction and its effects on behavior, relationships and lifestyle. Drug use as it relates to HIV transmission is presented with special emphasis on the sharing of needles and the use of bleach to sterilize injection equipment. Also stressed is the relationship between drug use, reduced inhibition and unprotected sex. Needle hygiene is discussed in relationship to self-esteem and self-caring. Harm reduction through the use of non-injected drugs is also discussed. Participants are asked to share their experiences of drug use and addiction, with discussion focusing on its negative consequences. Needle hygiene is taught and demonstrated using bleach, water and syringes. Participants rehearse these preventive techniques. Videotapes about HIV-infected IDUs are also shown to highlight the risk of HIV transmission through this route.

The final single-sex module is used to review and reinforce the information provided in the first three sessions, with an emphasis on identifying barriers and developing strategies for risk reduction. An AIDS personal risk assessment is self-administered as an exercise to help participants better assess their own drug- and sex-related risks.

Mixed-gender sessions are held on a weekly basis and serve two primary functions. First, the groups provide a forum for discussion of important life issues related to AIDS prevention, including homelessness, poverty, reproductive health, domestic violence, parenting and drug addiction. Our early experience with the project showed that these issues are often of greater immediate concern to high risk individuals than the somewhat abstract prospect of HIV infection and disease, and that it is critical to address change in sexual and drug use behavior as part of larger lifestyle issues. Secondly, the mixed-gender groups provide a forum for addressing the complex interpersonal issues around safer sex and safer drug use. For example, many women express reservations about initiating condom use because of the psychological threat of rejection by their partner, and because they may even fear that this could lead to violence or loss of financial support. Activities used to encourage men and women to talk to each other about these issues include group discussions, role playing and other experiential activities, and viewing and discussion of relevant videotapes. Presentations and discussion by persons with AIDS, recovering addicts and other role models are also a feature of the mixed-gender groups.

As shown in Figure 2, activities conducted in each stage of the intervention–street outreach, individual counseling and group sessions–relate directly to key aspects of the Health Belief Model and Social Learning Theory. All three stages of the intervention incorporate didactic education about HIV/AIDS and AIDS prevention, which, in addition to providing factual information, is intended to address issues of the salience of AIDS, perceptions of susceptibility to and severity of the disease, and perceptions of benefits and barriers to risk reduction. Both individual and group sessions incorporate exercises to assist participants to assess their own risk behavior, a more personalized approach to identifying benefits and barriers to risk reduction.

Manual skills training, a component of both individual and group sessions, is an experiential activity to increase perceived self-efficacy and decrease the perceived barriers to risk reduction, as well as to provide mastery of condom use and needle sterilization. Group sessions include training in the communication skills needed to negotiate condom use and to avoid needle sharing, again intended to increase self-efficacy and decrease the perceived barriers to risk reduction. Role playing exercises serve these same functions, and also provide experiences in which participants may begin to develop emotional coping responses to stressful interpersonal interactions related to risk reduction.

An exercise used in the group sessions specifically intended to increase self-efficacy is the setting of short-term, individualized, achievable goals by each participant (e.g., simply discussing condoms with a sexual partner). This is particularly appropriate when working with participants whose low self-efficacy expectations may be rooted in long personal histories of failed attempts to abstain from drug use or to make other desired life changes.

The long-term, group nature of the intervention design is intended to facilitate the creation of peer groups which can provide mutual reinforcement for adoption of a lower risk lifestyle, and to maximize opportunities for observational learning. This aspect of the intervention is reinforced by the recruitment of social networks of IDUs and crack users into the project, rather than simply recruiting isolated individuals. The use of credible role models, which include both multi-racial staff who are indigenous to the project's

FIGURE 2. RELATIONSHIP OF BEHAVIORAL THEORY TO INTERVENTION

DESIGN AND TECHNIQUES

INTERVENTION CHARACTERISTICS	INTERVENTION SETTING
Didactic Education about HIV/AIDS and Prevention	Outreach
	Individual Counseling
Affect beliefs about:	Group Sessions
severity	
susceptibility	
costs/benefits of behavioral change	
Increase saliency of AIDS prevention	
Personal Assessment of AIDS Risk	Outreach
	Individual Counseling
Identification of specific risk behaviors	Group Sessions
Identification of barriers to change	
Identification of benefits of behavioral change	
Manual Skills Training	Individual Counseling
	Group Sessions
Increase behavioral capacity/mastery of skills	
Increase self-efficacy	
Decrease perceived barriers to risk reduction	
Social/Negotiation Skills Training	Group Sessions
Increase self-efficacy	
Decrease perceived barriers/costs	
Use of Role-Playing	Group Sessions
Develop emotional coping responses	
Increase behavioral capacity/mastery of negotiation skills	
Decrease perceived barriers to risk reduction	

INTERVENTION CHARACTERISTICS	INTERVENTION SETTING
<u>Setting of Achievable Short-term Goals</u>	Group Sessions
Increase self-efficacy	
<u>Multiple Contacts with Participant</u>	Group Sessions
Repetition of information and skills rehearsal	
to increase self-efficacy	
Development of peer support:	
Observational learning of AIDS prevention behaviors	
Peer encouragement for AIDS prevention behaviors	
<u>Use of Credible Role Models</u>	Outreach
	Group Sessions
Affect beliefs about severity and susceptibility	
Increase self-efficacy	
Enable observational learning	

intervention areas and invited guests who are recovering addicts, also provide opportunities for observational learning.

DISCUSSION

Although using condoms and sterilizing injection equipment is technologically quite simple, the process by which individuals adopt safer sexual and needle use practices is not. Most theoretical and operational models for health promotion have not been developed to meet the special AIDS prevention needs of IDUs and crack cocaine users who are not in treatment settings. It is important that theories of health behavior change be refined and adapted to address the problems of this population, and that programs be developed which are accessible and acceptable to this hard-to-reach population. As Kelly et al. note ". . . AIDS high-risk behavior is probably determined by multiple cognitive, situational, self-control, social skill, and relationship factors . . . This argues in favor of multi-faceted prevention efforts" (1989, p. 66). We have drawn on key elements of two well developed theories, the Health Belief Model and Social Learning Theory, and attempted to operationalize these in a design that is appropriate to working with addicted individuals who are often justifiably suspicious and uncomfortable with health and social service providers.

There is a clear need for evaluation research to assess the efficacy of this and other AIDS prevention efforts targeting high risk drug users. Studies which shed light on the relative contributions of different aspects of the HBM and SLT to changing long-established sexual and drug use behavioral patterns are particularly important. Of obvious interest is the applicability of these and other health behavior theories to individuals whose cognitive abilities may be altered by drug use, and whose decision-making may be heavily influenced by the effects of extreme poverty, homelessness, violence and other characteristics of much of urban America. More information is also needed on how different theoretical constructs may best be operationalized when working with marginalized populations who lack regular contact with health and social service providers.

It is our hope that the project described here and similar efforts developed elsewhere may serve as models for AIDS prevention work with drug users in many different settings. However, it is important to note that this project has been developed independent from any existing healthcare setting. Philosophically, we have adopted a "harm reduction" approach, which focuses on AIDS prevention first, and promotes abstinence from drug use only secondarily. To the extent possible, our efforts are designed to help crack users and IDUs to incorporate safer sexual and drug use practices into their current lifestyles, rather than attempting more radical behavior change. Such an approach may well be difficult to implement in many clinical settings or drug treatment programs, and suggests the need either to develop independent, community-based AIDS prevention programs, or to rethink how harm reduction approaches might be integrated into the mainstream of the healthcare system.

REFERENCES

Bandura, A. (1977). Self-efficacy: Toward a unifying theory of behavioral change. *Psychological Review, 84*(2), 191-215.

Becker, M. H. (1974). (Ed.) The Health Belief Model and personal health behavior. *Health Education Monographs, 2*, 324-473.

Brown, L. S. & Primm, B. J. (1988). Sexual contacts of intravenous drug abusers: Implications for the next spread of the AIDS epidemic. *Journal of the National Medical Association, 80*(6), 651-656.

Centers for Disease Control (CDC) (1992, April). *HIV/AIDS Surveillance Report*. Washington, DC: U.S. Government Printing Office.

Chaisson, R. E., Osmond, D., Moss, A. R., Feldman, H. & Biernacki, P. (1987). HIV, bleach and needle sharing (letter). *The Lancet, 1*(8547), 1430.

Chitwood, D. D., McCoy, C. B. & Comerford, M. (1990). Risk behavior of intravenous cocaine users: Implications for intervention. In Leukefeld, C. G., Battjes, R. J. & Amsel, Z. (Eds.) *AIDS and Intravenous Drug Use: Future Directions for Community-Based Prevention Research*. National Institute on Drug Abuse, Research Monograph 93. Rockville, MD: U.S. Department of Health and Human Services.

DesJarlais, D. & Friedman, S. (1988). The psychology of preventing AIDS among intravenous drug users: A social learning conceptualization. *American Psychologist, 43*(11), 865-870.

Fisher, J. D. (1988). Possible effects of reference group-based social influence on AIDS-risk behavior and AIDS prevention. *American Psychologist, 43*(11), 914-920.

Iguchi, M., Watters, J., Biernacki, P., McCoy, C., Chitwood, D., Wiebel, W., Liebman, J., Kotranski, L., Williams, M. & Brown, B. (1990). Update: Reducing HIV transmission in intravenous drug users not in drug treatment–United States. *Morbidity and Mortality Weekly Report, 39*(31), 529, 535-538.

Jackson, J. F., Rotkiewicz, L. G. & Baxter, R. C. (1990). The role of drug abuse treatment programs in AIDS prevention and education programs for intravenous drug users: The New Jersey experience. In Leukefeld, C. G., Battjes, R. J. & Amsel, Z. (Eds.) *AIDS and intravenous drug use*: Future directions for community-based prevention research. National Institute on Drug Abuse, Research Monograph 93. Rockville, MD: U.S. Department of Health and Human Services.

Janz, N. K. & Becker, M. H. (1984). The Health Belief Model: A decade later. *Health Education Quarterly, 11*, 1-47.

Kelly, J. A., St. Lawrence, J. S., Hood, H. V. & Brasfield, T. L. (1989). Behavioral intervention to reduce AIDS risk activities. *Journal of Consulting and Clinical Psychology, 57*(1), 60-67.

Liebman, J., McIlvaine, D. S., Kotranski, L. & Lewis, R. (1990). AIDS prevention for IV drug users and their sexual partners in Philadelphia. *American Journal of Public Health, 80*(5), 615-616.

Liebman, J., Mulia, N. & Bowden, J. (1992). A model for AIDS education and counseling with intravenous drug users and their sexual partners. In: NOVA Research Company. (Ed.) Community-Based AIDS Prevention Among Intravenous Drug Users and Their Sexual Partner: The Many Faces of HIV Disease. Bethesda, MD: Author.

Liebman, J., Mulia, N. & McIlvaine, D. S. (1992). Risk behavior for HIV infection of intravenous drug users and their sexual partners recruited from street settings in Philadelphia. *Journal of Drug Issues*, 22(4), 867-884.

Magura, S., Shapiro, J. L. Grossman, J. I. & Lipton, D. S. (1989). Education/support groups for AIDS prevention with at-risk clients. *Social Casework: The Journal of Contemporary Social Work*, *1*, 10-20.

Mason, R. (1990). Fighting AIDS on the streets. *AIDS Education and Prevention*, 2(1), 84-88.

Mays, V. M. & Cochran, S. D. (1988). Issues in the perception of AIDS risk reduction activities by Black and Hispanic/Latina women. *American Psychologist*, 43(11), 949-957.

McAuliffe, W. E., Doering, S., Breer, P., Silverman, H., Branson, B. & Williams, K. (1987). An evaluation of using ex-addict outreach workers to educate intravenous drug users about AIDS prevention. Paper presented at the Third International Conference on AIDS. Cited in D. DesJarlais & S. Friedman (1988). The psychology of preventing AIDS among intravenous drug users: A social learning conceptualization. *American Psychologist*, 43(11), 865-870.

Mellinger, A. K., Goldberg, M., Wade, A., Brown, P. Y., Hughes, G. A., Lutz, J. P. & Harrington-Lyon, W. (1991). Alternative case-finding methods in a crack-related syphilis epidemic. *Morbidity and Mortality Weekly Report*, 40(5), 77-80.

Minkoff, H. L., McCalla, S., Delke, I., Stevens, R., Salwen, M. & Feldman, J. (1990). The relationship of cocaine use to syphilis and human immunodeficiency virus infections among inner city parturient women. *American Journal of Obstetrics and Gynecology*, *163*, 531-536.

Murphy, D. L. (1988). Heterosexual contacts of intravenous drug abusers: Implications for the next spread of the AIDS epidemic. *AIDS and substance Abuse*, New York: The Haworth Press, Inc.

Perry, C. L., Baranowski, T. & Parcel, G. S. (1990). How individuals, environments and health behavior interact: Social Learning Theory. In Glanz, K., Lewis, F. M. & Riner, B. K. (Eds.) *Health behavior and health education: Theory, research and practice.* San Francisco: Jossey-Bass.

Rhodes, F., Corby, N. H., Wolitski, R. J., Tashimi, N., Crain, C., Yankovich, D. R. & Smith, P. K. (1990). Risk behaviors and perceptions of AIDS among street injection drug users. *Journal of Drug Education*, 20(4), 271-288.

Rolfs, R. T., Goldberg, M. & Sharrar, R. G. (1990). Risk factors for syphilis: Cocaine use and prostitution. *American Journal of Public Health*, 80(7), 853-857.

Rosenstock, I. M. (1990). The Health Belief Model: Explaining health behavior through expectancies. In Glanz, K., Lewis, F. M. & Riner, B. K. (Eds.) *Health behavior and health education: Theory, research and practice.* San Francisco: Jossey-Bass.

Rosenstock, I. M., Strecher, V. J. & Becker, M. H. (1988). Social Learning Theory and the Health Belief Model. *Health Education Quarterly, 15*(2), 175-183.

Sorenson, J. L. (1991). Preventing HIV transmission in drug treatment programs: What works? *Journal of Addictive Diseases, 10*(4), 67-79.

Zweig, M., Singh, T., Htoo, M. & Schultz, S. (1990). *Crack use and congenital syphilis in New York City.* Poster presentation at the annual conference of the American Public Health Association.